Learning to care

on the

SURGICAL WARD

Moira Attree
MSc, BNurs, SRN, NDN, HV, RNT

Freelance Lecturer in Nursing

Jane Merchant
MSc, SRN, RCNT, DANS, RNT

Lecturer in Nursing, University of Manchester
Surgical Ward Sister, Manchester Royal Infirmary

HODDER AND STOUGHTON

LONDON SYDNEY AUCKLAND TORONTO

LEARNING TO CARE SERIES

General Editors

JEAN HEATH, MED, BA, SRN, SCM, CERT ED
National Health Learning Resources Unit,
Sheffield City Polytechnic

SUSAN E NORMAN, SRN, NDNCERT, RNT
Senior Tutor, The Nightingale School,
West Lambeth Health Authority

Titles in the series include:
Learning to Care on the Medical Ward
A MATTHEWS
Learning to Care in the Community
P TURTON and J ORR
Learning to Care for Elderly People
L THOMAS
Learning to Care in the A&E Department
G JONES
Learning to Care in Community Psychiatric Nursing
M WARD and R BISHOP

British Library Cataloguing in Publication Data
Attree, Moira
    Learning to care on the surgical ward.—
    (Learning to care series)
    1. Surgical nursing
    I. Title   II. Merchant, Jane
    610.73'677   RD99

    ISBN 0 340 38622 3

First published 1987
Copyright © 1987 M Attree & J Merchant

Typeset in 10/11 Trump Mediaeval by
Rowland Phototypesetting Ltd, Bury St Edmunds, Suffolk

Printed in Great Britain for Hodder and Stoughton Educational,
a division of Hodder and Stoughton Ltd, Mill Road, Dunton Green,
Sevenoaks, Kent, by Richard Clay Ltd, Bungay, Suffolk.

EDITORS' FOREWORD

In most professions there is a traditional gulf between theory and its practice, and nursing is no exception. The gulf is perpetuated when theory is taught in a theoretical setting and practice is taught by the practitioner.

This inherent gulf has to be bridged by students of nursing, and publication of this series is an attempt to aid such bridge building.

It aims to help relate theory and practice in a meaningful way whilst underlining the importance of the person being cared for.

It aims to introduce students of nursing to some of the more common problems found in each new area of experience in which they will be asked to work.

It aims to de-mystify some of the technical language they will hear, putting it in context, giving it meaning and enabling understanding.

PREFACE

This book is intended as a practical guide to the care of patients undergoing surgical procedures and is aimed at student nurses preparing for and during their first experience on a surgical ward. As part of the *Learning to Care* series, its purpose is to introduce the basic principles of planning patient care in specific settings.

The approach we have taken is different from most surgical nursing books. Basic human activities have been divided into groups and the pre-, peri- and post-operative aspects of the nursing care in these groups have been considered. In order to relate theory to practice and to remind students of the relationship between physical and psychosocial aspects of care, patient histories have been used to illustrate how the principles discussed in each chapter may vary when applied to actual people. Activities are suggested at the end of each main chapter to help you apply what you have learned to the patients on your own surgical ward.

Theory and practice in any discipline are closely related; nursing is no exception. Reference has been made, where possible, to nursing research to provide scientific support for the nursing actions suggested. Nursing also draws upon theories from the biological, physical and social sciences. These have not been discussed in detail; neither have we tried to provide a comprehensive guide to surgical procedures. Textbooks on these subjects will therefore need to be used in conjunction with this book and suggestions for further reading are provided.

This book focuses on the nursing responsibilities for assessing, planning and implementing patient care and *not* upon actual procedures or techniques. There is no substitute for practical experience; lessons are learned more readily and are longer lasting if they occur during the process of giving care under the supervision of an experienced nurse. During your time on the surgical ward, your goal should be to achieve a basic working knowledge and level of competence in the care of surgical patients.

The stated aims of this book are wide ranging and therefore not easy to accomplish in a single volume. We hope that this book will provide a starting point and stimulate interest upon which expertise can be built.

Acknowledgements. To Michael Attree, Dr Robert Attree and Mrs Hicks.

CONTENTS

The surgical ward

The major focus of nursing in a surgical ward is the care of patients undergoing and recovering from surgical (operative) procedures. A wide variety of operations may be undertaken, or the ward may specialise in one aspect of surgical care, such as abdominal or chest surgery. In spite of these variations the principles involved in providing nursing care for patients will be the same, or similar, on all surgical wards. It is these principles which you should try to learn when first working in a surgical area.

The majority of patients in a surgical ward will undergo some sort of operative procedure during their stay in hospital. Procedures may be extensive or quite minor and may be performed under anaesthesia or sedation. Some patients will be admitted to the ward for observation and investigations of a condition which is thought likely to need surgical treatment; for example, to ascertain the cause of abdominal pain. Not all of these patients will actually require an operation. A few patients who are admitted may be found to be unfit for anaesthesia, or it may be decided that their condition is unlikely to respond to surgery. Some are actually discovered, at the time of operation, to have diseases which cannot be surgically treated. The care of these patients, some of whom will not recover, is as important as that of patients who have successful operations, and will be discussed in Chapter 9.

Many patients arrive on the surgical ward as planned admissions from the waiting list. These patients have been referred by their

Anaesthesia Loss of sensation induced by drugs. *General* controllable and reversible state of unconsciousness, *local* localised loss of sensation without loss of consciousness.

I

General Practitioner to an Outpatient Clinic at the hospital because of symptoms or problems they have developed. If the surgeon believes that they would benefit from an operation, their names are placed on the waiting list and they are asked to come into hospital when a bed is available. In addition, some patients are admitted straight from the Outpatient Clinic because they require immediate treatment. Patients admitted to the ward as emergencies have usually been brought to the Accident and Emergency Department of the hospital or direct to the ward (often by ambulance) because of the sudden, or acute, development of symptoms which their General Practitioner believes require urgent treatment.

There will therefore be a wide variation in the physical condition of patients admitted to surgical wards. Those admitted from the waiting list will usually be quite fit but patients who are admitted as emergencies may be severely ill. Some patients may have pre-existing conditions, e.g. diabetes mellitus, which, although not the reason for their current admission, may affect their care.

The age range of patients in a surgical ward can be wide, although in most hospitals separate surgical wards are provided for children.

Various investigations are carried out on surgical wards. The most common are blood tests (to measure haemoglobin, red blood cells, white blood cells and electrolytes), and chest X-rays and electrocardiographs (ECG), which are usually carried out to ensure that patients are fit to have a general anaesthetic. In addition, special X-rays may be required, e.g. barium meal or intravenous pyelogram; and ultrasound or isotope scanning may be requested to aid diagnosis. The nursing staff may be asked to collect specimens for special tests (e.g. 24 hour urine collections; mid-stream specimen of urine; sputum; faeces). Nurses who have already worked on medical wards will be familiar with many of these tests. Patients may be admitted to the ward for investigations that need to be carried out under local or general anaesthetic, e.g. the removal of a small piece of tissue for examination under a microscope (a biopsy) or the internal inspection of an organ such as the bladder (a cystoscopy).

The pace of work on the surgical ward may appear to be extremely rapid. There is often a fast turnover of patients especially if the surgical ward is one which deals with a large number of minor procedures, which involve only one night in hospital or for which the patient is admitted as a 'day case'. On certain days, perhaps when there is a theatre list, or when a number of patients are being admitted from the waiting list, this may be very confusing. It is therefore not unusual for junior nurses to feel that it takes them some time to 'settle in' on a surgical ward.

Whatever the specialty of the surgical ward, the aims of care can be summarized in the following way:

1 to help the patient understand the surgery which is to be performed and its possible effects
2 to ensure that the patient is in the best psychological and physical state possible prior to surgery

Peri-operative
The period of time from the patient's transfer to theatre to his return to the ward.

3 to carry out preparatory procedures in order to minimize the risk of mistakes or complications occurring during the peri-operative period.
4 to prevent and/or detect any post-operative complications
5 to restore the patient to the maximum health and independence possible after surgery.

3

Teamwork is required in order to achieve these aims. Each ward usually has clerical and domestic staff as well as nurses, and sometimes specialist nurses are called upon (e.g. the stoma care nurse). The medical staff, who carry out the surgery and monitor the patient's medical progress before and after the operation, are headed by the consultant surgeon. Another doctor, the anaesthetist, usually visits the patient pre-operatively.

Various paramedical staff may be members of the team, commonly the physiotherapist and dietician, although others may be involved. For example, if you work in a surgical unit where some patients have a limb amputated, the physiotherapist and occupational therapist are key members of the team. The nurse should also remember that the theatre staff make a very important contribution to the care of surgical patients (Chapter 4).

Surgical ward team

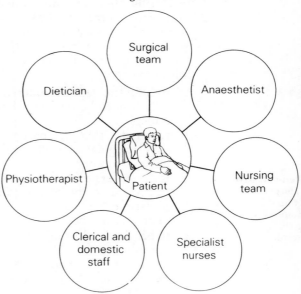

In addition there are other hospital staff who provide services which are required in order to give effective care to patients. These include the pharmacy, laundry, stores and equipment, laboratories, portering, catering and maintenance. The ward sister co-ordinates all these functions, ensuring the ward has adequate supplies and drawing together the particular team members required to help an individual patient.

The role of the nursing staff on the ward involves the observation and reporting of the patient's condition; assessing the needs of patients, planning and delivering the care required and evaluating the effectiveness of the care given. This process is summarized below.

Model of surgical nursing process

Admission/assessment
↓
Pre-operative preparation
↓
Peri-operative care
↓
Post-operative care and recovery
↓
Rehabilitation
↓
Discharge and follow-up

The Registered nurses in the ward team take the lead in this process and particularly in assessing the patient's needs and planning the care to be given. Assessment is not just carried out when a patient is admitted to the ward but is a *continuous* process because the condition of the patient is altering and therefore the care required may change rapidly. Although many patients are quite fit when admitted to the ward, they will become completely dependent when they have an anaesthetic and may only slowly return to independence after a surgical procedure.

After assessment of the patient's needs, an appropriate member of the nursing team is allocated to care for him. Junior nurses usually work alongside more senior nurses or are allocated to look after patients who require the sort of care they are familiar with. The nurses are then asked to report to sister/staff nurse about the care they have given and observations they have made. The more senior nurse helps to evaluate the effectiveness of nursing care given and the planning of continued care.

The principles of care for many of the patients in the ward may be similar, e.g. the preparation carried out pre-operatively to ensure the safety of patients undergoing surgery. There may be a tendency for nurses to see some of this care as 'routine'. If the majority of patients are undergoing the same type of surgery there may even be standard care plans or checklists to guide the nurses. It is important to remember that the experience of being admitted to hospital and having an operation is not 'routine' for the patient (or his family). Try to approach each patient as an individual, as it is possible for patients, especially those having 'minor' surgery, to feel that they are on a 'production line'. Admission to hospital, fear of the unknown and apprehension about surgery are all likely to provoke anxiety. It is part of the nurse's role to try to alleviate this anxiety (Chapter 3).

Learning to care for surgical patients

As a junior nurse you may find working on a surgical ward rather frightening at first. The care being carried out by the nurses may appear to be complex, e.g. special preparations for theatre and technical procedures such as the care of intravenous infusions and wound drains. This may be overwhelming at first but you will not be expected to have specialised knowledge and skills when you begin work on the ward. You should, however, take every opportunity to work with more experienced nurses and so observe procedures you are not familiar with.

Even the most inexperienced nurse can contribute to the care of patients by being thoughtful and helpful to patients, relatives and colleagues. Spend time talking to patients and carry out the care which is entrusted to you thoroughly. Record and report all your observations conscientiously and remember that *communication* (with patients and with other nurses) is probably the most important skill you can develop. Take every opportunity to observe and ask questions, but do not attempt to carry out any procedures you have not been taught. *Never be afraid to admit that you do not know something and to ask advice.*

Certain situations may be particularly worrying for nurses new to the surgical ward. Common fears are:

1 not understanding or not being able to carry out technical procedures
2 not knowing what to tell patients or relatives about the surgery or care of the patient if asked
3 not knowing what to do when patients have severe pain
4 not being able to cope in an emergency, e.g. a haemorrhage or cardiac arrest.

You will not be left on your own to cope with any of these situations and should always ask for guidance if you are unsure. For example, if a patient confesses to you his anxiety about a forthcoming operation and asks you questions about the procedure, you can explain that you are new to the ward and unable to answer his questions adequately. Assure him that you understand that this is very important to him and immediately ask the nurse in charge of the ward to deal with the patient's queries.

Many wards have specially designed teaching plans or objectives for students or your tutor may suggest objectives. If you do not have either you may find it helpful to use the following guidelines.

A   Familiarize yourself with the geography of the ward with special reference to patients' facilities (e.g. bathroom, dayroom) and sluice, kitchen and storage areas.

Learn the names of the members of the ward team; nursing, clerical and domestic. Learn the names of the patients you are asked to help care for.

Check the pattern of the usual day on the ward, e.g. meal times, visiting times, admission and operation days.

Ensure that you know where the resuscitation equipment is kept, what the emergency phone numbers are for fire and cardiac arrest and learn to use the oxygen and suction equipment.

Locate – the procedure and policy manual
       – the off duty rota and request book
       – the nursing Kardex or care plans
       – medical notes and X-rays.

B   Find out more about the type of surgery performed on your ward, ask questions and be prepared to do some reading to help your understanding.

Observe patients, listen to the ward report and examine care plans. You will find these a source of information to help you understand the care planned for the patients. You will also find that some of the care required is familiar to you and that you can make a contribution immediately. If you do not understand what is happening to a patient or the rationale behind any action you are asked to take, be sure to find out.

C   There will be certain knowledge and skills that you will need to acquire while working in the surgical ward. You may not have met these before and will need help to master them, e.g.

– pre-operative preparations
– care and maintenance of intravenous infusions
– care of nasogastric tubes and wound drains
– aseptic technique.

It is important initially to settle into the ward and become familiar with some of the basic principles of surgical nursing care. In this way you are making a contribution to the care of patients and will feel more relaxed and therefore able to acquire new skills and learn about the particular specialty you are working in.

The principles of surgical nursing will be covered in the following chapters. Specific examples related to patients will be used to illustrate these principles. Because there are many types of surgery the examples used may not relate to the patients you encounter on your first surgical ward. You should, however, find it possible to extract the principles from what you read. To help you, use the references for further reading and the questions at the end of each chapter.

FURTHER READING

Castledine, G. & McFarlane, J. 1982. *A Guide to the Practice of Nursing using the Nursing Process.* London: The C.V. Mosby Company.
Evans, D. M. D. 1981. *Special Tests and their Meanings.* 12th Ed. London: Faber and Faber.
Matthews, A. 1982. *In Charge of the Ward.* Oxford: Blackwell Scientific Publications.

2 Introduction to surgical patients

This chapter introduces five patients whose surgical histories are used throughout the book to illustrate how the nursing responsibilities discussed in each chapter may differ when applied to individual patients. Brief details of the operative procedures they undergo are provided. You are advised to consult other texts for full details of these and other surgical operations.

HISTORY

Julie Smith, aged 15 years is a schoolgirl.

Julie is admitted as an emergency on the request of her General Practitioner following a home visit. Julie's mother had become increasingly concerned that the abdominal pain Julie had complained of the previous evening had worsened over-night, preventing her from sleeping. In the morning, after drinking a cup of tea she vomited.

Julie was admitted to the ward at 2 p.m. accompanied by her mother. After taking a history and examing Julie, the doctors made a diagnosis of appendicitis, (an acutely inflamed appendix) and planned surgical removal (an appendicectomy). Pethidine 50 mg for pain and prochlorperazine 12.5 mg for nausea were prescribed intramuscularly. Julie's mother signed the operation consent form as Julie is under 16.

On admission Julie was experiencing lower abdominal pain, feeling nauseated, and wor-

Consent All adult patients must give their consent in writing for procedures and/or investigations to be carried out, after being given the relevant information. In the case of children this consent is given by a parent or guardian.

ried about the prospect of an operation as she had never been in hospital before and was not often ill.

Appendicectomy (removal of the appendix) is performed under general anaesthetic. Pre-operative preparation is usually minimal, involving the administration of a premedication and preparation of the abdominal skin as well as general pre-operative measures, e.g. withholding diet and fluids. An incision is made in the lower right abdomen through which the appendix is located, clamped and removed – a purse string suture is inserted around the stump and is pulled closed. The layers are repaired and the skin is sutured. A wound drain is not usually required. The wound heals quickly leaving no muscular weakness. Full activity can be resumed after 4–6 weeks. Sutures are removed on the 5th to 7th day usually by the community nurse as discharge is possible after 4 to 5 days if no complications occur.

HISTORY

Peter West, aged 35, is married with 2 young children. He is self employed and is a partner in a newly established small computer business.

Peter was admitted as a day case for a gastroscopy after being seen in the Outpatients Department. He was referred by his General Practitioner whom he had consulted after experiencing recurrent episodes of upper abdominal pain and severe indigestion. Peter's General Practitioner had discussed the possibility that he may have a peptic ulcer (erosion of the lining of the stomach or duodenum) which may be associated with irregular meals, high alcohol consumption and heavy smoking. On admission Peter expressed his anxiety about being absent from his business, and his inability to alter his lifestyle sufficiently to prevent his symptoms recurring. Peter is also anxious to know when the results might be available so that he can 'get sorted out' and be able to concentrate on his business.

Parts of the stomach

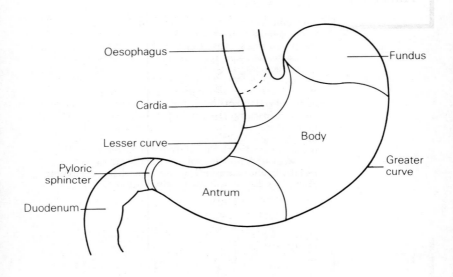

A gastroscopy is a diagnostic procedure involving the direct observation of the upper gastro-intestinal tract with a flexible fibre optic tube which is passed down the oesophagus. Air is introduced into the stomach to distend it for easier visualisation. A small specimen of tissue can be taken for examination through a biopsy channel. The procedure is usually carried out under intravenous sedation and a local anaesthetic, and takes approximately 15 to 30 minutes to complete. It can be uncomfortable but is not painful.

Preparation involves the withdrawal of diet and fluids 6 hours pre-operatively, and post-operatively until the effects of the local anaesthetic have worn off – approximately 1 hour. Observations for signs of perforation of the oesophagus or stomach, e.g. severe abdominal pain, should be made.

The patient can go home when he feels able. Results of the gastroscopy can be discussed with the patient before discharge and treatment can be prescribed. The patient is asked to attend the Outpatients Department for the biopsy results which can take 7–10 days. Advice regarding diet and smoking is given prior to discharge.

Mrs Mary Fellows, aged 45, is married with two children aged 13 and 15. She is a part-time shop assistant and a housewife.

Mrs Fellows consulted her General Practitioner 8 months ago after noticing that the veins in both legs were becoming increasingly prominent, her legs ached and her ankles became swollen. She had also noted patches of discoloured skin on the inner aspect of both ankles which itched. Her General Practitioner referred her to the surgical Outpatients Clinic where the surgeon examined her and placed her on the waiting list for stripping (removal) of varicose veins. He also advised her that there would be a delay of some months before she was admitted and strongly advised her to reduce her weight by 10 kg and to try hard to stop smoking prior to admission.

Mrs Fellows was admitted to the ward the day before her planned surgery. She had reduced her weight from 81 to 74 kg – still above the recommended level for her height 1.6 metres (5'3"). She had managed to reduce her cigarette consumption initially but started again when the letter arrived asking her to come into hospital.

Varicose veins are abnormal dilations of the veins due to stasis and back pressure, often caused by incompetent valves, weak walls of the vein and exacerbated by increased pressure from above, e.g. obesity, pregnancy. Common sites are the short and long saphenous veins of the leg.

Stripping and ligation of varicose veins involves the insertion into the vein of a long flexible tube with a head at one end (a 'stripper'), which is pulled through and out at the groin incision tearing the vein from the surrounding tissue. Haemorrhage is avoided by the application of pressure from the toes upward as the 'stripper' passes. The entry and exit wounds are sutured and any deep perforated veins are located and tied off (ligation). The procedure is performed under general anaesthesia. The skin is usually prepared pre-operatively by removing any hair which is present.

For the first 24 hours post-operatively the foot of the bed is elevated to 45° to aid venous return. Mobility is promoted gradually. Recovery is usually uneventful and discharge is possible within 1 to 2 days. Sutures are usually removed in the groin after 5 days and in the leg at 7 days.

Deep veins of the leg

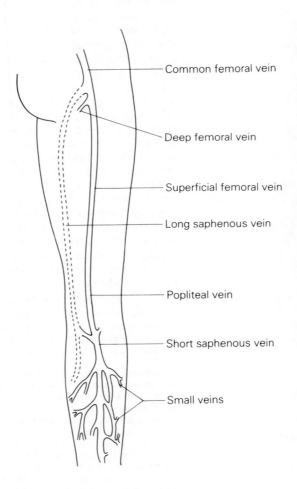

Common femoral vein

Deep femoral vein

Superficial femoral vein

Long saphenous vein

Popliteal vein

Short saphenous vein

Small veins

Mr Harry Reynolds, aged 65 years, is a retired furniture shop manager.

Mr Reynolds is admitted directly from the surgical Outpatient Clinic where his General Practitioner referred him urgently because of his history of an alteration in bowel habit, rectal bleeding and constipation. He arrives accompanied by his wife. Mr and Mrs Reynolds appear bemused by the speed of events and do not seem to be aware of the severity of the situation, despite a discussion with the surgeon about the possibility of the need for a colostomy (a surgically formed opening into the colon through which faecal material is excreted).

The surgeon requested urgent investigations, a barium enema (X-ray of the colon) and sigmoidoscopy (direct observation of the colon) with biopsy of the rectal mass; and preparation for surgery. The surgeon had already informed Mr and Mrs Reynolds of the possibility that an abdomino-perineal resection of rectum may be required. Mr Reynolds was understandably shaken; even though he had 'suspected the worst' (cancer), he had not expected such an extensive operation. He had never been in hospital before and consulted his General Practitioner infrequently.

Mr Reynolds will require a great deal of psychological as well as physical preparation for surgery.

An abdomino-perineal resection of rectum is a major operation, taking 2–4 hours. It usually involves 2 surgeons working simultaneously; one working in the abdomen removing the colon and performing a colostomy and the other working on the perineum removing the rectum and anus. Due to the development of an instrument which can staple the ends of the rectum together lower than was previously possible, fewer abdomino-perineal resections now need to be performed.

Extensive preparation of the gastro-intestinal tract is required to ensure the bowel is free from faecal matter. Potential post-operative problems include pain, shock, haemorrhage and infection. Recovery is often slow in the early stages. Management of the colostomy has to be learnt before discharge and the patient may stay in hospital for 10–14 days post-operatively.

Colon and rectum

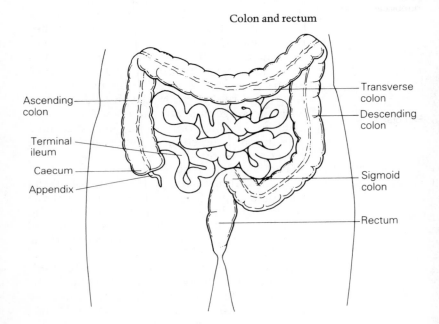

HISTORY

A hernia is a protrusion of part or the whole of an internal organ or organs through its normal coverings. The most common variety occurs at sites of weakness in the abdominal wall.

Mr William Brown, aged 75 years, is a retired post office worker. He is widowed and now lives alone in a ground floor flat in a warden controlled sheltered housing scheme.

Mr Brown has been having increasing pain and a 'dragging' sensation in his right groin. There is now quite a large lump in his groin which his General Practitioner diagnoses as an irreducible right inguinal hernia. He refers Mr Brown to the Outpatient Clinic where the consultant arranges to admit him to hospital promptly, because of the risk of strangulation.

Mr Brown is in fact admitted to hospital 10 days later for repair of his hernia.

Common hernia sites

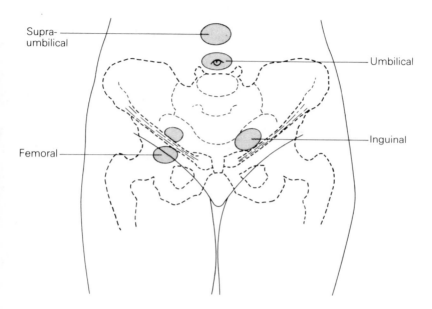

Supra-
umbilical

Umbilical

Femoral

Inguinal

An *inguinal hernia* occurs at the point where nerves, blood vessels and the spermatic cord (in males) pass through the lower abdominal wall. An irreducible hernia may strangulate, i.e. the contents of the sac of the hernia may be constricted so that the circulation is cut off, thus leading to gangrene and eventually perforation of the bowel (a surgical emergency).

A hernia is repaired by returning the contents of the sac (usually a loop of bowel) into the peritoneal cavity, excising the sac of the hernia and repairing the muscle wall by suturing. This operation usually requires only a short stay in hospital of 3 or 4 days.

You will meet these patients again in the following chapters and may find it helpful to refer back to this chapter to refresh your memory when reading about them.

ACTIVITIES

1 Read more about the surgical procedures mentioned in this chapter and ensure you understand them before reading on. The

staff on the surgical ward may suggest useful references. Talk to your tutor or clinical teacher who should be able to recommend helpful books in your library.

FURTHER READING

Rowett, H. C. Q. 1983. *Basic Anatomy and Physiology.* 2nd Ed. London: John Murray (or a textbook of anatomy recommended by your School of Nursing).

A textbook of surgery recommended by your School of Nursing.

3 Stress, anxiety and pain

Stress and Anxiety

The term anxiety is often used to describe the emotional reaction of an individual to a stressful event such as entering hospital. Like other terms associated with emotional states, stress is difficult to define and varies from person to person. It has been implicated as a causative factor in both psychological and physical disease. In surgical wards you will often have to care for people who display anxiety. For the purposes of this chapter we will define anxiety as an emotional state usually involving fear, tension and apprehension and commonly associated with anticipation of a threat. For patients in surgical wards, fear of the unknown and anticipation of unfamiliar and possibly painful procedures will probably be the commonest causes of anxiety.

The experience of admission to hospital and the possibility of surgery will be different for each individual but it is possible to discuss some of the physical and psychological factors which may contribute to stress and the effects these may have on progress and recovery. This chapter will suggest contributions you may make towards minimizing patients' possible anxiety.

Many patients may not feel able to express their fears and it is therefore important to recognise other signs of anxiety. These include excessive pallor or flushing of skin; rapid, darting eye movements; perspiration; tremor of hands; rigid posture; aggressive manner; ex-

cessive and/or irrelevant talking, and not looking directly at the person being spoken to.

Pain

Pain is a difficult concept to define because
each individual experiences it differently. It is
both a biological and a psychological experience and is influenced by factors such as age,
sex, personality and previous experience and
expectations. Because of the subjective nature
of the experience, pain tends to be enhanced by
anxiety and stressful situations. A good definition of pain is:

> 'Pain is whatever the experiencing person
> says it is and exists whenever he says it
> does.'
> *McCaffery*, 1972

When you are working in a surgical ward
you should remember that although the operation performed may give you some indication
of the pain a patient is likely to experience,
there will be a great variation in practice. Some
of your patients will have pain when they
come into hospital, others will only experience pain post-operatively.

The relationship between anxiety and pain

Research evidence suggests that where anxiety
can be relieved pre-operatively, patients are
likely to experience less pain after surgery.
Adequate psychological preparation is also
thought to reduce the incidence of post-
operative vomiting and complications and in
some cases the length of stay in hospital. Since
all information given to patients may not be

retained or understood, you must try to give information clearly and concisely, check patients' understanding, offer patients opportunities to ask questions and be prepared to repeat information when necessary.

Because of the close relationship between anxiety and pain they will be considered together in the remainder of this chapter.

Admission

For most people admission to hospital, whether planned or as an emergency, is a traumatic event. It may be difficult for hospital staff to remember this because they are familiar with the environment and routines. The individual entering hospital as a patient, whether for the first time or not, will be leaving behind his usual environment and lifestyle. Try to remain aware of the factors which may make a newly admitted patient anxious. For example, these may include pain, discomfort, nausea or other symptoms which may be distressing. There may be apprehension about being in hospital and the surgery itself and sometimes fear about prognosis and/or dying. Lack of privacy, loss of security and personal identity and isolation from family and friends may also contribute to anxiety.

You will find that even when you are very new to the surgical ward, you can contribute to reducing the effect of some of these factors by simple strategies such as introducing yourself by name to new patients and offering your help while they adjust to their new situation. A welcoming manner to both patients and relatives is one important way in which feelings of strangeness and isolation can be minimized. Including relatives (or friends) in this and offering information such as visiting times and the hospital telephone number reassures the patient that there is no intention of cutting him off from his family and social contacts.

Each new patient is assessed by the nursing staff soon after admission so that care can be planned, taking into consideration the particular needs of the individual. A member of the nursing staff usually discusses in detail the patient's lifestyle and the effects on this of his present illness and admission to hospital. This discussion should always be a two-way exchange of information, during which the patient should feel free to ask questions and express fears. At this time the nurse may find it possible to gauge whether the patient is anxious and if so what the source(s) of this anxiety may be. The relationship formed between the nurse and the patient is therefore extremely important and a few simple measures will help ensure that a patient feels relaxed enough to discuss things fully. For example, the nurse should make time to talk to the patient and not be involved in other

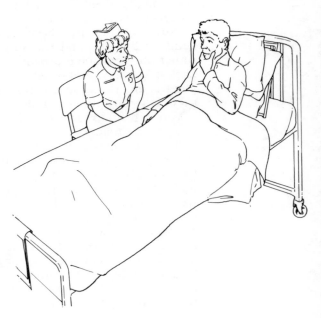

activities which might distract her. Both the patient and the nurse should be seated comfortably and some effort should be made to ensure privacy. If there is no room in which interviews can be conducted, the nurse and patient should be seated near to each other so that they can converse quietly. Tactfully expressed, open-ended questions will need to be used to obtain maximum response from the patient.

The depth of information obtained at this interview will depend upon the custom in your ward, the time available, the relationship between the nurse and patient, the nature of the condition affecting the patient and the type of admission. For example, it may be the practice on your ward to obtain less information from patients who are admitted as day cases than those who are to stay in hospital for some time and often it is not practical to conduct any sort of interview with someone who is admitted as an emergency.

Consider the example of Julie Smith (Chapter 2). It is clearly inappropriate to involve Julie in a prolonged conversation as soon as she arrives on the ward. In this case, the priorities are comfort, information and preparing Julie safely for her operation.

Julie was made comfortable in bed and given a vomit bowl and tissues as she continued to feel nauseated. It was explained to her that she should not drink prior to having an anaesthetic but she was given a mouthwash because her mouth felt dry. When asked she said that she would like her mother to stay with her and would prefer the nurse to obtain any necessary information from her mother.

The pre-operative period
The length of the pre-operative period will vary from patient to patient. In the case of Julie Smith it will be very short and admission

procedures, nursing assessment and preparation for theatre will have to be compressed into a very short space of time.

HISTORY

The doctor explained the nature of the operation to Julie and her mother and they both agreed that it was necessary. Mrs Smith signed the consent form because Julie was under 16 years of age. The nurse then came to prepare Julie for theatre. An identity bracelet was put on her wrist with her full name and hospital record number written on it. Julie had bathed on the previous evening and in view of this and her discomfort it was agreed that shaving and skin preparation would be carried out in theatre. She was given a clean theatre gown and was then allowed to rest until the theatre porter arrived to collect her. The nurse who had been looking after Julie escorted her to theatre and stayed with her until she had been introduced to the theatre nurse.

For non-emergency patients the time between admission to hospital and surgery will be at least 24 hours. This allows time for the patient to settle in hospital, for nursing and medical staff to complete their respective (psychological and physical) assessments of the patient and for investigations and special preparations to be carried out.

During this time patients will also require information about the peri- and post-operative periods. This ensures that anxiety is not exacerbated by fear of the unknown.

Summary of information patients will require
1   Day and time of operation.
2   Physical preparations required and reasons for them, e.g. shaving, bathing.
3   The procedure immediately prior to operation, e.g. whether premedication will be given.

4   What should be expected post-operatively,
    e.g. if the patient will wake up in the ward
    or a recovery room; whether to expect an
    intravenous infusion.
5   What relatives should do about visiting or
    telephoning on the day of operation.

Some of this information you will quickly
learn and will feel able to discuss with
patients, but other items (e.g. what to expect
after a particular operation) you may not know
enough about. In some units theatre staff visit
patients to help with this. *If patients ask
specific questions which you cannot deal with
you should always refer this to sister.*

HISTORY

When Mr Reynolds (Chapter 2) arrived on the
ward he was quiet and withdrawn. He was
accompanied by his wife who was flustered
and appeared to have been crying.

NURSING CARE

Mr and Mrs Reynolds provide an example of
the need for nursing care which is planned to
alleviate anxiety and distress. They need to be
greeted in a welcoming manner and would
perhaps be helped by being offered a cup of tea
and time to talk quietly together. Later it
would be helpful if both were given an opportunity to talk to the ward sister and doctor.

Mr Reynolds will be in hospital for some
days prior to surgery and so there is no need for
either the medical or nursing assessments to
be made immediately.

When Mr Reynolds talked to a nurse later in
the day, he expressed the following concerns:

– He was very worried about the rectal bleeding and believed that the consultant's decision to admit him so quickly indicated his
  condition was serious.
– He understood very little of what was said to

him in the Outpatient Clinic and could not explain it to his wife.
- He anticipated his wife's distress and knew that she 'feared the worst'.
- He was embarrassed about the nature of his illness and reluctant to discuss his bowel function with anyone, especially young women.
- He was pleased that he and his wife had been able to talk to the doctor but he was still not sure that he understood about either the X-rays of his bowel or the surgery which might be necessary.

The nurse, aware of these fears, should be continuously alert for opportunities to offer support and aid understanding.

During the pre-operative period Mr Reynolds will also have several investigations performed, including a barium enema and a sigmoidoscopy and biopsy. He will require preparation of his bowel for these and will therefore need explanation of the preparation as well as the procedures.

In addition Mr Reynolds will eventually undergo major surgery on his bowel and will have a colostomy raised. Physical preparations are required for this (Chapter 4, 5 and 6) but psychological preparation is equally important. Formation of a stoma requires the patient to change his usual bowel habit. This is distressing and is likely to change the patient's body-image and is a threat to the person's usual lifestyle. Preparation for this type of surgery may be shared with the stoma care nurse and/or the patient may sometimes be introduced to someone who already has a stoma. A teaching plan may be devised for the patient and the information needed may be given in short sessions so that the patient has time to absorb the information and ask questions.

Sigmoidoscopy is the passage of a rigid lighted instrument into the rectum and sigmoid colon to examine the mucosa or take a biopsy.

Stoma From Greek word meaning 'mouth' and 'opening'. In surgery used to describe an artificial opening to divert urine or faeces.

Body-image The mental image an individual has of his own body (including emotional attitudes and values).

On the first occasion Mr Reynolds met the stoma care nurse he was very quiet and seemed reluctant to discuss anything. She talked to him for only a short while and left him a booklet with clear diagrams of the proposed surgery. He read this and showed it to his wife and on the following day asked questions.

The stoma care nurse and ward nurses were able to answer his questions over the next few days and also showed Mr Reynolds some of the bags which can be worn over a stoma and let him practise handling these. Finally, shortly before the operation, the stoma care nurse marked the site on his abdominal wall where the stoma would be sited (the consultant may sometimes do this).

Mr Reynolds was also given information about the operation and what would happen to him afterwards so that he knew what to expect. He remained anxious about the surgery and its outcome but felt that he understood what was happening to him.

The post-operative period
In the initial post-operative period patients may be drowsy from the effects of anaesthesia or analgesia. Many will therefore appear relaxed and sleepy but some may not remember much of what they were told pre-operatively and may experience disorientation, alarm, pain or occasionally confusion.

Nursing responsibilities
1 To assess the patient's emotional and physical state, including signs of post-operative shock (Chapter 5) and pain and to report these.
2 To carry out nursing procedures designed to enhance physical and psychological comfort, e.g. lifting or moving into a comfortable position; orientating the patient or answering questions.
3 To carry out medical instructions, e.g.

controlling the flow of an intravenous infusion; giving analgesics or anti-emetics prescribed and monitoring their effects.

At first the nurse may be totally responsible for the physical care and well-being of patients who may be unable to carry out their normal activities. Although this varies a great deal from patient to patient, all post-operative patients are likely to have some degree of anxiety and/or pain.

HISTORY

Julie was awake when she was collected from the recovery room and was distressed by the sensation of being lifted from the theatre trolley into bed. Once in bed she felt unable to move at all and became tearful. It was explained to her that her wound was the source of the discomfort and she was given an intramuscular injection of pethidine 75 mg. Sister explained to her that this could be repeated when necessary.

Discharge
Many surgical patients will have anxieties about leaving hospital. For example, they may be concerned about the surgical wound, when they should recommence work, whether the condition will recur or whether they will make a full recovery.

HISTORY

Peter had a gastroscopy performed under local anaesthetic and returned to the ward immediately afterwards. He was told that he would be allowed to drink in one hour's time when the local anaesthetic had worn off and he was able to swallow. He would then be allowed home. He was most anxious to know the result of his investigation and whether the cause of his pain could be treated without his having more time off work.

Peter has a duodenal ulcer which can be treated with drug therapy. Before Peter leaves the ward the doctor explains to him the regime of drugs which are to be prescribed. He also talks to him about the possible relationship between stress, smoking, poor dietary habits, alcohol and the incidence of peptic ulcers so that Peter understands what is happening and can consider what changes he might make in his lifestyle.

Peter is also given an appointment with the dietician for advice and an appointment at the Outpatient Clinic to enable the medical staff to monitor his progress. He tells sister that he is relieved to know that his illness is treatable but is not sure how to change his lifestyle. Sister discusses with him the possibility of getting help from his General Practitioner and also points out to him that there may be support groups in his locality for people who wish to give up smoking or classes to learn relaxation techniques which may be helpful.

Peter's situation illustrates the fact that patients who spend very little time in hospital or have minor procedures performed still have anxieties and may need a great deal of help both before and after discharge.

Anxieties about going home and resuming activities may appear more obvious to the nurse when a patient has had major surgery. Mr Reynolds for example will need a great deal of preparation for discharge. Even at the time of his admission and immediately prior to surgery when he has been given a great deal of information, his overriding concern is how he will cope with a stoma and whether he will be able to manage at home.

Intensive pre-operative teaching and preparation will help prepare Mr Reynolds for the process of learning how to adapt to life with a stoma. The rehabilitation process may take quite a long period of time and will involve giving the patient enough support to boost his confidence and promote independence. Mrs Reynolds will need to be involved in this process in order to help relieve her anxieties and so that she can also support her husband.

The stoma care nurse has already assured Mr and Mrs Reynolds that she will visit them when he leaves hospital and that the ward staff will also arrange for the district nurse to give help should it be necessary.

ACTIVITIES

1 Next time a patient is admitted to your ward for 'planned' or 'routine' surgery, observe all the things which you think may be a source of anxiety and list them.
2 What strategies can a nurse use to relieve a patient's anxiety on admission to hospital?
3 Choose two patients on your ward, one having major and one minor surgery. List the information you think each patient will require before going to theatre and why you think the information is needed.

FURTHER READING

Bridge, W. & Macleod Clark, J. 1981. *Communication in Nursing Care*. London: HM & M Publishers.
Boore, J. R. P. 1979. Nursing surgical patients in acute pain. *Nursing*, 1st series, **1**, 37–43.
Hayward, J. 1975. *Information – A Prescription Against Pain*. London: RCN.
McCaffery, M. 1972. *Nursing Management of the Patient with Pain*. Philadelphia: J. B. Lippincott Company.
Wilson-Barnett, J. 1979. *Stress in Hospital*. Edinburgh: Churchill Livingstone.

4 Safety in the surgical ward

Adults are usually able to meet their own safety needs. Exceptions to this are people who are mentally or physically disabled or those who are developmentally immature and are therefore unaware of dangers to themselves or are unable to protect themselves from hazards. This includes people with hearing or visual defects who may not hear or see danger.

Many people admitted to hospital will still be able to protect themselves from most hazards but it is the responsibility of the nurse to assess the patient's ability to do this. There will be times when all patients undergoing surgery will be unable to look after their own safety needs; that is when they are immobilized, sedated or anaesthetized.

You should also remember that you too have safety needs and you should learn about potential dangers to yourself and other staff. These include hazards which may cause injury like poor lifting techniques or wet floors, and those which may cause infection for example infected materials such as blood or faeces, soiled linen, used needles or knife blades.

You will be taught about hazards both in the classroom and on the wards and should always adhere to procedures and policies laid down for the safety of patients and yourself.

Environmental hazards

Potential hazards in the hospital environment are numerous. They include wet and/or slippery floors; trolleys and furniture on wheels which may move if brakes are not applied; equipment blocking corridors and gangways, and wires left hanging between furniture or across floors. All these may cause falls. Patients, especially those with poor vision or mobility, are most at risk but so are staff and visitors to the hospital.

Soiled dressings and linen and poorly cleansed equipment are all sources of bacteria. Patients in hospital are more susceptible to infection than most people, particularly those with wounds, the very ill and those receiving steroid or immunosuppressant drugs. Staff however are also at risk and items such as broken glass, unsheathed needles and used knife blades may cause infection (particularly hepatitis) as well as injury.

Other potential sources of injury in hospitals may be faulty electrical equipment, excessively hot water (especially to patients with poor sensation or those who are confused) and excessive exposure to X-rays.

Nursing responsibilities
1 To be aware of possible hazards in your ward area.
2 To be aware of and adhere to policies (e.g. for patient safety; for disposal of refuse).
3 To assess whether patients are at risk for any reason and to minimize any risk to them.
4 To inform senior nursing staff and/or appropriate departments about risks (e.g. electricians about faulty sockets).

Radio-active implants A source of energy placed in the body which emits electromagnetic waves used to treat malignant cells locally.

The list of hazards given above is not exhaustive. In addition you may work in a specialized unit where there are particular hazards that you must learn about, for example where implants of radio-active materials are used. Such special units have their own procedures for dealing with these hazards. *Remember that if you are unsure about any-*

thing which may have a safety implication you should ask sister or staff nurse.

Personal safety of patients

Remember that some patients will be more prone to hazards than others but that there may be occasions when all patients could be at risk.

Admission

This is the time when patients are assessed and nurses have an opportunity to decide whether a patient has particular problems which could endanger personal safety. The sort of problems that might put a patient at risk are restricted mobility; poor/no vision; poor hearing; severe pain, vomiting or diarrhoea; and serious illness especially if the patient is in a very debilitated state.

HISTORY

Arthritis is a painful condition characterized by inflammation of a joint or joints.

Chronic bronchitis is an inflammation of the bronchi which is present over a long period of time.

NURSING CARE

When Mr William Brown was admitted to the ward for repair of his hernia he was quite relaxed. He had been in hospital many years before to have his appendix removed and that had been an uneventful procedure. He said that he would be relieved to have the operation performed because his hernia was now bothering him a great deal. He complained that it reduced his ability to walk around which was already somewhat restricted by arthritis. He also noticed that the hernia became larger and more painful when he coughed. At times this was very difficult for him because he had chronic bronchitis and therefore coughed a great deal.

The nurse who assessed Mr Brown decided that his arthritis and the hernia were causing him pain, restricting his mobility and might endanger his safety. This was discussed with Mr Brown and as a result he was given a variable height bed which could be kept low to enable him to get in and out easily. His bed was also within easy walking distance of the toilet and bathroom so that he could remain independent and active without being in danger of falling or of tiring himself excessively (see also Chapter 8).

His chronic bronchitis was also noted as this might make him unfit for anaesthetic or at risk of a post-operative chest infection as well as exacerbating his present problems. The decision about his fitness for anaesthesia would be made by the medical staff. The nurse also notified the physiotherapist about Mr Brown's problems (see also Chapters 5 and 8).

During the assessment interview there should be a two-way exchange of information so that the nurse gives information to the patient about procedures which are designed for his safety, and answers questions.

At this time certain information is usually recorded to ensure the patient is fit for surgery and also to avoid potential complications, e.g. a specimen of urine is tested to ensure that diabetes mellitus does not go undiagnosed; allergies are checked to ensure that drugs, anaesthetic agents, lotions or dressings can be avoided if a patient has an allergy to them. Temperature, pulse, respiration, blood pressure and weight are also recorded. This is also related to patient safety and reasons for this are discussed in Chapters 5 and 6.

Pre-operative period
The aim of pre-operative care is to prepare the patient both physically and psychologically for surgery. This means that the nurse must understand what hazards the patients may be exposed to and what peri- and post-operative

complications may occur. The nurse's responsibility is then to prepare the patient for theatre in such a way as to avoid and/or prevent these whenever possible. The prevention of stress and anxiety has already been discussed in Chapter 3.

Nursing responsibilities

1 Explain tests and procedures to the patient to help reduce anxiety.
2 Record baseline observations.
3 Assist with any tests required to ensure patient is fit for anaesthetic.
4 Help to teach breathing and leg exercises.
5 Offer information about post-operative events.
6 Reduce skin bacteria by:
   – shaving proposed wound site or using depilatory cream (if it is the policy of the unit)
   – ensuring hair, nails and umbilicus are clean
   – carrying out any specific skin preparation requested (e.g. painting skin with antiseptic lotion).

You may work in a ward where specific preparation is required in addition to this, e.g. to ensure that the bowel is clear (Chapter 6).

Near to the time of operation specific measures are carried out to safeguard patients. These are usually supervised by a qualified nurse and must be carried out so that they meet the requirements of law and hospital policy.

CHECKLIST	*Aim*	*Nursing Action*
	The patient will be psychologically prepared for surgery	– ensure the patient has assimilated all information given – offer opportunities to ask questions – explain all procedures

Aim	Nursing Action
The correct patient will receive the correct operation and legal requirements will be met	– check patient has a correctly completed identification band
	– check consent form has been signed
	– check patient's notes, X-rays and results of investigations available
To ensure correct pre-operative preparation has been carried out	– ensure pre-operative fasting (4 hours minimum) has been adhered to
	– check any special preparations are complete (e.g. bowel preparation)
	– ensure all skin preparation complete
	– help patient change into theatre clothes (according to hospital policy)
	– change bedlinen
To prevent incontinence of urine and ensure ease of access in pelvic surgery	– ask patient to empty bladder
To ensure no loss of property and reduce risk of injury to patient (e.g. from diathermy burns; or from inhaling loose objects)	– valuables stored and recorded if necessary
	– jewellery and hair pins removed
	– if wedding ring left on cover with hypo-allergic tape
	– prosthesis removed (e.g. false teeth) or noted (e.g. dental crowns) NB. Hearing aid is usually left in position until patient anaesthetised to aid communication
To ensure anaesthetist can check patient's colour	– remove all cosmetics and nail polish
To ensure rest, reduce anxiety and dry secretions	– administer premedication as prescribed (and to conform with law and hospital policy)
To avoid risk of patient falling	– ask patients not to get out of bed after premedication and instruct in use of call system

Aim	Nursing Action
To give patient continued psychological support until anaesthetised	– nurse who has been caring for patient escorts him to theatre and hands over to theatre nurse.

You will remember that Julie Smith was admitted for an emergency appendicectomy and was only in the ward for a short period before going to theatre. Pre-operative preparation was therefore limited to the essentials (Chapter 3). Mr Reynolds however was in hospital for over a week before having an operation to remove a carcinoma from his bowel.

NURSING CARE

During the first few days that Mr Reynolds was in hospital the main aims of his care were to confirm the diagnosis of carcinoma of the rectum, and to ensure that both Mr and Mrs Reynolds understood the implications of this. It was also important to ensure that Mr Reynolds was fit to undergo surgery and to prepare him both physically and psychologically for the operation.

To assess Mr Reynolds' fitness, various observations (temperature, pulse, respirations, weight, urine tests) and routine blood tests were carried out and checked to ensure that the results were within normal limits. Blood was cross-matched and was in fact needed for a transfusion prior to surgery because Mr Reynolds was found to be anaemic. In addition, a routine chest X-ray and ECG were performed.

Anaemia A deficiency in the quality and/or quantity of red blood cells.

A barium enema and a sigmoidoscopy and biopsy of the rectal mass were required to confirm the diagnosis of carcinoma of the rectum. Both of these were uncomfortable procedures and required explanation to Mr Reynolds and preparation of the bowel.

In order to clear the bowel for the investigations, Mr Reynolds had a low residue diet and then a period of time before each investigation where his intake consisted only of fluids. Because he had already lost some weight and had been found to be anaemic the dietician was consulted to ensure that he received adequate nourishment.

Prior to each of the investigations and the operation, Mr Reynolds was given an enema and then rectal washouts. These removed the residue of barium and all faeces and ensured a clear view for both the investigations and the operation. They also minimized the risk of infection caused by faecal matter accidentally spilling into the peritoneal cavity during the operation. Antibiotics were also prescribed for 48 hours prior to the operation to reduce the bacteria normally present in the bowel.

During this time Mr Reynolds was taught breathing and leg exercises by the physiotherapist to prevent post-operative complications and the stoma care nurse, together with the ward nurses, taught him about having a colostomy and caring for it.

Mr Reynolds often looked tired and anxious during the days preceding his operation and it was important that the ward nurses gave him opportunities to ask questions and express his fears and also ensured that he had time to rest.

During the 24 hours prior to surgery the house officer explained the operation again to Mr Reynolds and ensured that he understood what was to happen before he signed the consent form. Clear fluids only were offered by mouth and during the evening a final rectal washout was given to ensure Mr Reynolds' bowel was clear.

When Mrs Reynolds came to visit her husband, the staff nurse spent some time with them both explaining what they should expect immediately after the operation and she arranged for Mrs Reynolds to telephone the ward the following afternoon.

In the evening abdominal and perineal shaves were carried out and Mr Reynolds then had a bath.

On the morning of the operation, Mr Reynolds was allowed nothing to eat or drink (for 6 hours prior to the scheduled time for the surgery). Each procedure to be carried out was explained and Mr Reynolds understood that the measures being taken were to ensure his safety. He bathed again and the stoma care nurse then marked the proposed site for the stoma on his skin. His bedclothes were changed and a nurse helped him into a theatre gown.

All the routine checks were then carried out (see Checklist pp. 35–37) before Mr Reynolds was given his premedication. He was then able to sleep for about half an hour before being taken to theatre. A ward nurse accompanied Mr Reynolds as far as the anaesthetic room, taking with her all his notes and X-rays to ensure that the surgical team had all the available information.

Peri-operative period
A ward nurse or member of the theatre staff remains with the patient until he is anaesthetized – this is for the safety and reassurance of the patient. Once a patient is sedated or anaesthetized he is completely unable to care for himself and he is dependent upon the theatre team to ensure his safety. The theatre nurse is part of this team and will help with the following:

– Ensuring that the correct operation is carried out for each patient.
– Assisting the surgeon to prevent hazards during the operation, e.g. infection, loss of swabs or instruments, burns from diathermy equipment.

Diathermy Very high frequency electric current used to coagulate the blood vessels or dissect tissues.

– Assisting the anaesthetist to monitor the patient during anaesthetic and recovery to prevent complications to breathing and circulation.

Post-operative period

Whether recovery from anaesthetic takes place in a recovery unit or surgical ward, the monitoring of the patient's condition to prevent complications is a nursing responsibility supervised by qualified staff.

All nurses must understand the principles involved in order to safeguard patients. The key nursing responsibilities involved in immediate post-operative care can be summarized as follows:

1   Oxygen, suction and emergency equipment must be at hand and in working order.
2   A nurse must remain with the patient to ensure a clear airway until the patient is conscious and the cough reflex has returned.
3   Communication must be effective between theatre and ward staff to ensure that ward nurses understand the nature of the surgery performed, the condition of the patient and the continuing treatment prescriptions.

Vital signs are temperature, pulse, blood pressure, respiratory rate.

4   The condition of the patient must be monitored (particularly the vital signs) to ensure that any post-operative complications can be quickly dealt with.
5   The patient must be kept comfortable and his continuing safety needs met.
    When the patient is conscious he should be reorientated and explanations and information offered.

The staff nurse collected Mr Reynolds from the Recovery Unit. He was conscious but still drowsy and his vital signs were stable. She obtained the following information and instructions:

– An abdomino-perineal resection of the rectum had been performed. There were two wounds; one abdominal and one perineal with a tube drain in place draining into a bag. Mr Reynolds had an intravenous infusion and a central venous line (see p. 52) and fluids had been prescribed for both.
– A nasogastric tube had been passed.
– A urinary catheter had been inserted and was draining into a sealed drainage system.

The following instructions were given:
– To monitor vital signs and measure the central venous pressure, half hourly at first.
– To aspirate the nasogastric tube 2 hourly.
– To measure urinary output hourly.
– To observe both wounds and drainage.
– Nothing to be taken by mouth.
– Analgesic and anti-emetic drugs had been prescribed.

During the next few days, until the patient can take over some aspects of care himself, nurses are responsible for his care and in particular for his safety. Patients may be unaware of some hazards (e.g. the possibility of developing deep vein thrombosis) and the nurse must therefore explain both the hazards and the preventive actions which can be taken. For example, when Mr Reynolds has fully recovered from his anaesthetic, he is still at risk from the possible complications of surgery. These complications and the nursing care required to prevent them is discussed in detail in other chapters. A list is given here as a reminder:

Deep vein thrombosis The formation of a blood clot in the deep vessels of the lower limb, usually as a result of pressure or stasis.

Paralytic ileus
Absence of
peristalsis in the
bowel leading to
abdominal
distension, nausea
and vomiting.

**Pulmonary
embolus**
Obstruction of the
pulmonary artery
or one of its vessels
by a travelling
blood clot.

Septicaemia
Systemic infection
of blood by
pathogenic
micro-organisms.

Shock and haemorrhage
Under- or overhydration
Pain
Nausea and vomiting
Paralytic ileus
Chest infection
Urinary tract infection
Deep vein thrombosis and pulmonary embolus
Pressure sores
Wound infection
Septicaemia
Inability to rest/sleep.

Rehabilitation and discharge

The role of the nurse involves ensuring the patient's safety while he regains independence and adapts to change in functioning or lifestyle, e.g. an amputee requires special help and teaching to achieve independence and learn new methods of mobility. This may also involve the help of the physiotherapist and occupational therapist. If the nurse neglects this part of her role the amputee may fall and injure himself or lose confidence in his ability to adapt and cope with this problem. A major part of the nurse's role is therefore to assess how much help a patient requires and what risks there may be to his safety. You may need help and advice at first but will gradually learn how to assess these factors.

The aim of this period of rehabilitation is to prepare the patient for discharge home and recommencing life in the community. It may be quite difficult to ascertain the conditions a patient will go home to and whether there are any risks involved. The ward nurses will need information from the patient and his family and from other people who may be involved with helping him in the community. Sometimes a home visit is planned, for example by the physiotherapist, in order to make a realistic assessment. The aim is to ensure that no patient is sent home to a situation where he might be at risk.

ACTIVITIES

1 Look around your ward and list any potential hazards – to staff, patients or visitors. Find out what policies there are to minimize these risks.
2 When you are assessing a patient who is being admitted to your ward, make a list of potential risks which may affect this particular individual.
3 Are any special preparations carried out before patients in your ward go to theatre? If so, what preparations are carried out and why?
4 Are any post-operative observations or procedures carried out in your ward that have not been mentioned in this chapter? If so, find out why these are necessary.

FURTHER READING

Saving lives. *Nursing*, 1st series, **14**, June 1980.
The Royal Marsden Hospital 1984. *Manual of Clinical Nursing Policies and Procedures*. London: Harper and Row.

5 Problems relating to breathing, circulation and shock

Breathing

It would help your understanding to revise the anatomy and physiology of respiration before proceeding with this section.

Living cells require a constant supply of oxygen and the removal of carbon dioxide to function. Any prolonged interruption to this process is a threat to survival; brain cells become damaged after two to three minutes without oxygen.

Respiratory tract

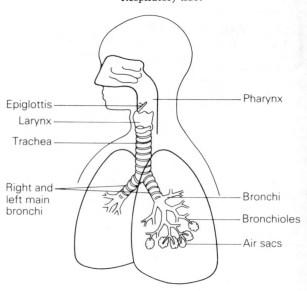

Epiglottis

Larynx

Trachea

Right and left main bronchi

Pharynx

Bronchi

Bronchioles

Air sacs

Maintenance of this essential process depends upon:

1 a sufficient oxygen supply
2 the ability to obtain and absorb oxygen
3 a system of transport for the oxygen
4 the ability to utilize the oxygen.

Surgery can interfere with all of these processes either directly, by operations on or near the heart and lungs, or indirectly via anaesthetic gases and drugs. Most surgical patients, regardless of the extent of their operation, are at risk of some degree of problem with breathing.

The patient's pre-operative condition can indicate the likelihood of breathing related problems arising post-operatively. The nurse's assessment should reveal potential problems amenable to nursing action, whilst the doctor's history, examination and investigations check for other problems such as chest infection or bronchitis, which can be dealt with medically before surgery. When surgery is planned there is time to correct existing problems and reduce the risk of potential problems.

The site of the proposed surgery also provides an indication of possible problems. Surgery near the lungs or involving muscles associated with respiration can affect breathing, for example. The pain following removal of the gall-bladder (situated close to the diaphragm) often makes patients reluctant to breathe deeply thus making them susceptible to chest infection.

Surgery on the heart or lungs themselves, or involving opening the chest for access (e.g. to the oesophagus) directly affects function, as air enters the normally airtight pleura, causing the lung to collapse. Re-inflation is achieved by removing the air through an underwater seal drain (chest drain). Following surgery to the heart or lungs, or any operation requiring a long period under anaesthesia, some patients fail to regain the ability to breathe independently and require mechanical assistance. This type of care is usually carried out in special units. You may however see a chest drain on a general surgical ward. *As a junior nurse it is important that you receive extra instruction and practice under supervision before caring for these patients.*

The nurse's main responsibilities with regard to breathing are set out in the following pages.

Admission

Observe and record the patient's respiratory rate, noting the rhythm, character and any breathing difficulties (e.g. wheeze, cough, sputum, pain). Check whether the accessory muscles of the chest and abdomen are being used during respiration.

Cyanosis The bluish appearance of skin and mucous membranes due to inadequate oxygenation.

Observe the skin and mucous membranes for pallor or cyanosis. Ask if the patient has a history of lung disease. Establish whether the patient smokes cigarettes or a pipe, the amount of tobacco taken daily and whether attempts have been made to give up or reduce consumption. If previous attempts have been unsuccessful, offer advice and encouragement to help the patient stop smoking during the pre-operative period.

Nursing responsibilities
1   Check for signs of chest infection (pyrexia or a productive cough). A sputum specimen may be sent for culture if an infection is suspected.
2   If a cough is present steam inhalations may be prescribed to help loosen secretions.
3   Check for items which may dislodge and be inhaled, e.g. loose or crowned teeth.
4   Refer patients to the physiotherapist who will assess each patient and teach them

deep breathing exercises to improve respiratory efficiency.

5 Encourage patients' mobility to aid circulation of oxygen to the tissues but ensure adequate rest to conserve energy for healing.

Pre-operative period

Withhold food and fluids for a minimum of 4 hours to prevent regurgitation and inhalation of stomach contents. If a premedication is prescribed it is usually administered between $1/2$ hour and 1 hour prior to the planned operation time. This may include anticholinergic drugs to dry up secretions and prevent inhalation of saliva. Sometimes sedatives or analgesics are given (e.g. morphine or diazepam). As some of these drugs depress the respiratory centre in the medulla, the premedicated patient should be observed closely for alterations in the respiratory pattern.

Anticholinergic drugs inhibit the passage of parasympathetic nerve impulses.

Peri-operative period

In theatre
The ward nurse may be asked to remain with the patient until fully anaesthetized. The patient's respiratory function is carefully controlled and monitored by the anaesthetist throughout the patient's stay in theatre. After the operation has been completed the anaesthetic will be reversed and the patient's normal control over respiration re-established.

On the ward
Prepare the equipment for the patient's return and ensure that it is functioning correctly. This will usually include oxygen, tubing and masks; suction, catheters and gloves and a post-anaesthetic tray containing tongue forceps and an airway. Resuscitation equipment should be nearby.

Pillows (to position the patient in order to maintain a clear airway) and equipment and charts for recording observations of vital signs are also prepared.

Post-operative period

Most respiratory complications, in particular obstructed airway, occur within 24 to 48 hours after surgery. A patient who is not fully conscious should never be left alone and an experienced nurse should accompany the patient back to the ward from theatre. Even though the patient may be fully recovered from the anaesthetic, he is still in danger.

CHECKLIST

Post-operative maintenance of airway
- Place the patient in the semi-prone (recovery) position.
- Keep the jaw well forward, support the angle of the jaw with your thumb. An oro-pharyngeal airway may be used.
- Keep the patient's head lower than chest to prevent fluid flowing into trachea.
- Change the patient's position two hourly to encourage secretions to drain from the chest and to relieve pressure on the chest wall.
- Ensure an adequate fluid input to prevent secretions becoming too viscous (thick and sticky). Suction may be needed to remove secretions.
- Administer oxygen if prescribed (usually humidified to prevent drying up of the mucus and paralysis of the protective cilia).

Observation and assessment

It is necessary to monitor the type and rate of respirations post-operatively. The frequency of this monitoring will depend upon the extent and type of surgery. A senior nurse will help you to assess the condition of the patient, decide how frequently observations should be recorded and plan appropriate nursing care.

You must report a respiratory rate lower than 12 per minute, a tachypnoea or any abnormality, such as wheezing or noisy respirations which might be caused by an obstructed airway. While observing the respiratory rate you should check whether both chest walls move equally and whether the accessory muscles of

Tachypnoea
Raised respiratory rate.

respiration are being used. It is also important to check the mucous membranes and lips for signs of cyanosis.

As consciousness returns
Observation of the patient's respirations will gradually be decreased if they are giving no cause for concern. The patient may gradually be raised until he is propped in an upright sitting position to reduce the pressure of the abdominal organs on the diaphragm.

You may encourage the patient to perform deep breathing exercises to aid oxygenation and to prevent stasis and infection in the lower lobes of the lungs. Gentle movement in bed also aids the circulation of oxygenated blood. When the patient is fit enough these measures are best performed as frequently as every 15 minutes.

The patient may need assistance to cough. It may be helpful if you support the wound while the patient is coughing to reduce discomfort and strain on the wound. A sputum pot and tissues should be provided if appropriate and steam inhalations may be ordered.

The physiotherapist should be informed of the patient's return to the ward so that she can assist with these activities. Pain experienced by the patient should be assessed regularly and analgesia given as appropriate, in particular prior to physiotherapy so that the patient feels comfortable enough to cough and breathe deeply, thus ensuring the maximum effect from physiotherapy.

It is important to assist the patient to change position regularly while in bed and to encourage ambulation as quickly as possible to assist the circulation. An upright posture in bed or chair also aids lung expansion.

Mr Brown was assessed as being at risk of post-operative chest complications due to his pre-existing bronchitis. He was treated pre-operatively by the physiotherapist who taught him deep breathing exercises. The nurses also encouraged him to drink 2 litres of fluid a day and gave him steam inhalations every 4 hours. His temperature and respiratory rate were within normal limits pre-operatively.

Despite the pre-operative precautions Mr Brown developed a moist-sounding cough post-operatively. His temperature rose to 37.8°C and was therefore monitored every 4 hours. His respiratory rate varied between 22 and 24 per minute.

The physiotherapist visited Mr Brown post-operatively and treated his chest. A sputum specimen was obtained and sent to the laboratory for analysis. The results showed that an infection was present which was sensitive to ampicillin. Steam inhalations were given four hourly and Mr Brown was given analgesia prior to physiotherapy. This treatment and the prescribed antibiotics started to take effect and after 4 days Mr Brown's temperature returned to normal levels and his chest sounded clear.

Circulation and Shock

You will find it useful to revise the anatomy and physiology of circulation and body fluids before reading this section.

Maintenance of an adequate circulation to provide the means of transport for oxygen and carbon dioxide depends not only on the correct functioning of the heart and vessels but also on the presence of an adequate amount of fluid to circulate.

The most common post-operative circulatory problem is shock. This can be defined as a

Simple diagram of circulatory system

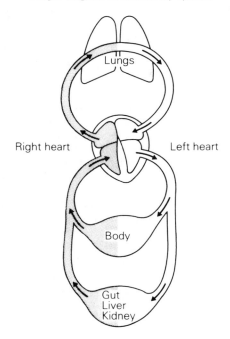

state of circulatory collapse which leads to low arterial blood pressure and oxygen shortage in the tissues. *Primary* shock occurs at the time of surgery, *secondary* more than 24 hours after surgery. If undetected and untreated, shock represents a major threat to survival.

Shock occurs to varying degrees in all surgical patients, due to alterations in the normal control mechanisms of the body. The medical history, examination and tests should check for pre-existing problems which can be corrected. These investigations involve haematological tests, ECGs, chest X-rays and blood grouping and cross-matching in case a transfusion should be required.

Effective pre-operative preparation and early recognition by close post-operative observation and prompt treatment can reduce the severity of shock.

Haemorrhage is one of the major causes of post-operative shock. Any blood or fluid loss reduces circulatory volume and thus oxygen-carrying capacity. Unless blood volume is restored, oxygen starvation occurs in the tissues leading to circulatory failure to the vital organs, and death follows. The body's natural reaction to reduced blood volume is to constrict peripheral blood vessels which leads to pale, cold and often clammy skin. The rate of heart contractions increases in an attempt to preserve blood flow to the vital organs. The effect of reduced blood volume to the brain is an alteration of conscious level – restlessness, irritability and sometimes aggression. These symptoms may be difficult to recognize in a patient after anaesthesia.

Reduced blood flow to the kidneys leads to oliguria (reduction in urine volume and thus increased concentration). Any tissue starved of oxygen increases its carbon dioxide production and the lungs compensate by deep and sighing respirations. Nursing observations are crucial in the early detection of shock. The patient's normal vital signs (pulse, blood pressure, respiratory rate and temperature) are established in the pre-operative period and variations 10% above or below the pre-operative measurement should be reported immediately.

If a patient is deeply shocked, measurement of peripheral blood pressure may be very low or difficult to record. Blood supply to the vital organs can be more accurately measured by a central venous pressure line. A line is fed through a peripheral vein until it reaches the right atrium of the heart. This is connected to a manometer. The manometer readings provide the best guide to circulatory volume and thus allow fluid replacement therapy to be accurately calculated.

You may come across central venous pressure lines on a general surgical ward. *Extra instruction and practice under supervision will be required before you will be able to care for patients with central venous pressure lines correctly.*

Fluid and electrolyte balance

For each cell to function correctly, the concentration of electrolytes and the amount and distribution of body fluids needs to be maintained within narrow limits. Fluid loss is usually accompanied by electrolyte loss. Either can cause cellular damage, impairing function and hindering recovery.

All surgical patients are at risk of disturbances in their fluid and electrolyte balance due to the effect of trauma and stress on the body. Pre-operative preparations to reduce the risk are very important, as is the correction of any pre-existing problem.

For clarity, fluid and electrolyte problems are considered separately.

Fluid Balance

In health, fluid intake is usually balanced with output. The body's response to alterations in fluid balance varies according to the rate and volume of fluid loss, the effects being more apparent when loss is rapid or when the patient is already debilitated. Fluid balance is an extremely delicate indicator of health and as such, can warn of serious problems much more quickly than pulse and respiratory rates. The accurate recording of fluid balance is therefore of vital importance. Problems of fluid balance can occur rapidly in surgical patients. Prevention of problems is preferable but not always possible, so early recognition and treatment is crucial.

1 Excess fluid loss will lead to dehydration which is dangerous to surgical patients as it predisposes to, and exacerbates, hypovolaemic shock (low circulatory volume). It may be caused by:

a) inability to take or absorb fluids, e.g. comatose patient
b) over-long pre-operative restriction of fluids
c) excessive fluid loss – vomiting, diarrhoea, haemorrhage, gastric suction, wound drainage, perspiration.

Anuria
Suppression of urine formation, in surgical patients due to reduced blood supply to the kidneys.

It is characterized by tachycardia, hypotension, pyrexia, anuria, dry cool inelastic skin, muscle weakness, depressed mental state.

Treatment is usually fluid replacement, prescribed intravenously unless oral fluids are indicated. All fluid output needs to be accurately measured and recorded including wound drainage and nasogastric aspirate and vomitus.

2 Fluid excess may occur in the postoperative period, and presents problems if the excess fluid is retained within the cells or in the vital organs as central and pulmonary oedema. It may be caused by:

a) over-rapid infusion of intravenous fluid
b) retention of sodium and therefore fluid.

It is characterized by tachycardia, hypertension, tachypnoea and shortness of breath, raised urine output, irritability, confusion, weakness and apathy.

Treatment usually involves withholding fluids, and stopping any infusions. Other medical measures may be indicated.

Electrolyte Balance
Electrolytes are inorganic substances dissolved in body fluid. The principal body elec-

trolytes are sodium, potassium and hydrogen ions. As electrolytes are acid or alkaline, disturbance of their delicate balance will affect body function.

Electrolyte imbalances are usually rare in surgical patients who were in good health pre-operatively and undergoing straightforward operations of relatively short duration. Patients who have pre-existing problems or who are undergoing major operations, in particular on the gut or urinary tract may, however, develop problems in the post-operative period. The main causes of electrolyte loss or excess in surgical patients are summarized in the following table:

Causes of electrolyte loss	*Causes of electrolyte excess*
i) loss of body fluid 　– diarrhoea and vomiting 　gastric aspirations 　leakage from 　wound/fistula.	i) excessive input, e.g. over addition of potassium to infusion solutions.
ii) increased urinary output.	ii) decreased urinary output.
iii) poor filtration by diseased kidney.	iii) poor filtration by diseased kidney.
iv) the effects of shock.	

In practice the clinical features of electrolyte imbalance are difficult to differentiate from other post-operative effects. The symptoms of electrolyte imbalance which the nurse may observe include:

1　tachycardia and/or irregular pulse
2　hypo/hypertension
3　changes in respirations
4　changes in mental state or behaviour, e.g. restlessness, irritability, apathy, lethargy – leading to coma
5　muscle weakness, spasm or cramp.

In order to determine the cause of the patient's problem it is usual for the doctor to send specimens of blood and sometimes urine to the laboratory pre and post-operatively for the measurement of electrolyte concentrations. *It is important that the nurse reports her observations of the patient's condition so that electrolyte disturbances are detected early and treated.*

Acid base balance

Hydrogen is one of the body's main electrolytes; its concentration (pH) in blood and body fluids needs to be maintained within a range of 7.37 to 7.45. For optimum cell functioning, blood pH is usually 7.4. A pH above 7.5 is described as alkalosis and a number below 7.3 is termed acidosis. Alkalosis and acidosis can result from problems with the regulation of respiration or metabolism and may therefore occur as a result of the effects of anaesthesia, the surgical procedure, fluid imbalance during the peri-operative period or a pre-existing condition, e.g. diabetes mellitus. The table below presents the causes and effects of acidosis and alkalosis.

Causes of acidosis
Respiratory: hypoventilation
Metabolic: diarrhoea,
bowel fistulae,
diabetic ketosis

Causes of alkalosis
Respiratory: hyperventilation
Metabolic: vomiting,
excessive gastric
aspiration, over diuresis,
excess infusion of sodium
bicarbonate

Effects of acidosis
Increased repiratory
force and depth
Tachycardia or arrhythmia
Diuresis
Lethargy: reduction in
consciousness leading
to coma

Effects of alkalosis
Slow, shallow respirations
Increase in body temperature
Cardiac arrhythmia
Increased diuresis
Muscle twitching

Admission

It is important to observe the patient's skin for signs of circulatory failure. Are the hands, nail beds and feet pink and warm? Do the patient's lips and tongue appear blue? Pulse and blood pressure are also important indicators of circulatory status.

Signs of fluid imbalance may sometimes be observed. For example, oedema of dependent parts suggests fluid excess, while dry, wrinkled skin and a dry tongue suggest fluid deficit. You should also establish the patient's usual pattern of fluid intake and output by tactful questioning.

Height and weight should be measured during the assessment. Once a baseline has been established daily weighing is the best guide to fluid gain or loss (1 litre of water weighs 1 kilogram). Alternatively, all fluid intake and output may be measured and recorded.

A specimen of urine should be requested and urinalysis performed including the estimation of urine specific gravity to assess fluid balance and renal function.

Pre-operative period

Encourage activity to improve the circulation and try to minimize stress as this exacerbates shock (see Chapter 4). If problems have been identified during assessment, monitoring of vital signs and fluid balance may continue. It may also be necessary to correct any fluid or electrolyte imbalance.

The effects of preventive and corrective measures will be monitored and the operation may be postponed until any problems have been resolved.

Immediately prior to surgery, fluid withdrawal should be kept to a minimum to reduce the risk of dehydration. You should check that the patient understands the pre-operative fluid restriction and the reason for it. If a fluid balance chart is in use it will be continued until the patient goes to theatre and will be one of the documents which accompany him.

Peri-operative period

Circulatory function will be monitored and maintained by the anaesthetist. It is normal for blood pressure and pulse rates to fall due to the effect of anaesthetic drugs and gases on the cardiac and respiratory centres. These effects may last for 3–4 hours post-operatively. Theatre staff usually wait until the patient's vital signs are stabilizing before allowing the patient to return to the ward.

Shortly after anaesthesia an intravenous infusion may be commenced to provide a route for fluid replacement. If blood loss during operation has been excessive, previously cross-matched blood will be transfused. When the nurse collects the patient from theatre it is important that she checks the patient's circulatory and fluid status and ensures that prescriptions for the fluid regime have been completed.

Post-operative period

During the time the patient is in the care of the theatre staff, preparations should be made on the ward for his return (see page 47). In addition special equipment may be required to assist in the maintenance of correct fluid balance, e.g. for an intravenous infusion, bladder drainage, nasogastric aspiration or surgical drains.

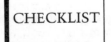

CHECKLIST

– Monitor and record the vital signs, reducing the frequency as the patient's conditions stabilizes.
– Note and report any indications of haemorrhage or shock, i.e.:
  – excessive bleeding via wound or drains
  – decreasing volume and rising rate of pulse
  – fall in blood pressure readings
  – fall in temperature and cold, clammy skin

- decrease in volume and increase in respiration rate
- decrease in urine volume.
NB. Central venous pressure may also be recorded.
- Follow all post-operative instructions, e.g. regulate any intravenous infusion.
- Accurately measure and record all fluid input and output (including vomit, nasogastric aspirate, urine, wound drainage).
- Carry out measures to prevent shock, such as keeping the patient warm and relieving pain.

NURSING CARE

Mr Reynolds' pre-operative assessment revealed no respiratory or circulatory problems apart from iron-deficiency anaemia, for which he received a blood transfusion. He was, however, thought to be at risk of developing post-operative complications because of the nature of the surgery to be undertaken. His condition was therefore monitored and he was prepared carefully for surgery. His pulse and blood pressure were recorded regularly and he was encouraged to drink at least 2 litres of fluid a day. He was weighed daily and a fluid balance chart was completed to check his fluid balance status.

Fluids were withheld completely for 4 hours prior to surgery but Mr Reynolds was adequately hydrated and passed urine before his premedication was given.

When he was fully anaesthetized both an intravenous cannula and a central venous line were introduced to give fluids and measure central venous pressure during the procedure. A nasogastric tube and a urinary catheter were also passed.

Mr Reynolds eventually returned to the ward after 5½ hours. He had been observed for some time in the recovery unit as his central venous pressure and blood pressure were low. He had lost blood during the operation and had required a replacement transfusion of 4 units of blood.

Mr Reynolds was collected by the ward staff

nurse who was told about his operation and progress and given instructions for his continuing care. He was taken back to the ward on his bed and staff nurse then checked his condition. His central venous pressure and blood pressure remained low but stable; there was a minimal amount of blood loss from the abdominal wound; 200 ml of fluid had drained via the perineal drain; 100 ml of urine were present in the urine drainage bag and Mr Reynolds was warm and comfortable.

During the next 12 hours observations of Mr Reynolds' vital signs were gradually reduced in frequency as they became stable and returned almost to pre-operative levels. All fluid input and output was carefully monitored. Post-operative instructions about the aspiration of the nasogastric tube and infusion of fluids were carried out.

Mr Reynolds was kept comfortable by lifting and moving him gently every 2 hours and giving him regular analgesia. Anti-embolic stockings were fitted to help prevent deep vein thrombosis. Mr Reynolds was kept warm and each procedure was quietly explained to him before it was carried out.

ACTIVITIES

1 Observe the physiotherapist working with patients in the pre- and post-operative period.
2 Select a patient who has difficulty breathing in the post-operative period. What measures were planned to help resolve the problem?
3 Select one patient who smokes and one who does not. Observe for any differences in their pre- and post-operative breathing patterns.
4 Select a patient who is depleted of fluid and one who has fluid excess. What are the

similarities and differences in their pre-
and post-operative care?
5   What post-operative observations would
indicate that a patient is developing shock?

FURTHER READING

Breathing: part 1. 1979. *Nursing*, 1st series, No. 6.
Breathing: part 2. 1979. *Nursing*, 1st series, No. 7.
Fluids in the balance. 1980. *Nursing*, 1st series, No. 13.
Intravenous therapy. 1982. *Nursing*, 2nd series, No. 7.
Circulation. 1984. *Nursing*, 2nd series, No. 26.
Breathing. 1984. *Nursing*, 2nd series, No. 27.
Breathing. 1984. *Nursing*, 2nd series, No. 18.

6 Problems relating to nutrition and elimination

Nutrition

Food is essential to human life because it supplies the energy required by living cells for maintenance, repair and activity. The definition of food can include both solids and liquids which provide sources of energy.

Most students will be familiar with the constituents of a well-balanced diet:

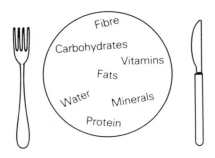

Your physiology book or a text on dietetics will provide all the information you need about these substances, their sources and how they are used by the body.

We spend much of our time buying food, planning meals and eating them. Eating is also a matter of habit and social activity and may have cultural or religious significance.

The specific amounts of nutrients required will vary at different stages in life (e.g. children need food for growth) and will vary with activity and state of health. However, a *well-balanced diet* is always required.

Factors a nurse should bear in mind when assessing a patient's nutritional needs:

Age	Condition of mouth/dentition
Sex	Ability to ingest food/fluid
Weight	Elimination
Usual activity/ occupation	Specific disease/condition
General health	Special diet (if prescribed)
	Any drugs prescribed

Tactful questioning is required and the nurse should avoid questions which imply criticism, e.g. questions about breakfast suggesting the patient *should* eat breakfast. Asking the patient to recall a typical 24 hours eating pattern is often the most helpful way of assessing dietary habits.

An individual's diet may vary for many reasons and while starvation is unusual in the Western world because of the availability of food, it is still possible for people in the West to suffer from inadequate nutrition.

Poor nutrition can be caused by inadequate or restricted intake of food for a variety of reasons. For example, dietary preferences, cultural and religious beliefs, ignorance of the availability or value of food items, or inability to obtain and prepare food. The latter may be due to inability to shop or cook, for example because of limited mobility or language problems. Poverty may cause people to eat less or cut out more expensive foods. Sometimes there may be mechanical or physiological problems which prevent the ingestion or digestion of food (e.g. ill-fitting dentures, diabetes mellitus).

It is important that a patient is well-nourished prior to surgery, as this helps the promotion of wound healing, resistance to infection and ability to overcome trauma. All stress (including anxiety and surgical trauma) increases the body's need for nutrients, particularly protein and vitamins. Any patient who has been unable to eat or who has lost weight may therefore require extra nutritional supplements before surgery. The ideal post-operative diet contains all the essential nutrients and is high in protein and vitamins.

Problems of nutrition and hydration
Some common problems you may come across are listed below:

Problem	Some causes
Inability to chew food	– no teeth – disease of mouth, tongue or jaw
Dysphagia	– foreign body or lesion in oesophagus
Nausea/vomiting	– pregnancy – fear/anxiety/pain – conditions of stomach or bowel
Anorexia	– pain – malignancy – gastro-intestinal disturbance
Inability to absorb/utilize food material or fluid	– diarrhoea – disease of bowel, e.g. Crohns disease

Dysphagia Difficulty with swallowing

Anorexia Loss of appetite.

In addition, medical and nursing interventions may lead to (or exacerbate) disturbance of nutrition and fluid and electrolyte balance. For example, admission to hospital may be a cause of anorexia, probably due to fear, anxiety, new routines and different foods and mealtimes. Also, treatment may require the restriction of food or fluid (for tests, X-rays or operations). The administration of anaesthesia or drugs, or procedures such as the preparation of the bowel for X-rays or surgery may also require restriction of the diet or affect appetite.

Nursing responsibilities

1　Assessment of the state of nutrition and hydration on admission and also the effect of admission and treatments.

2　Giving help and assistance to patients to overcome any problems defined during assessment (together with family, doctor and/or dietician).

3　Recording and reporting dietary and fluid intake when requested.

4　Participating in the administration of alternative methods of nutrition/hydration, i.e. parenteral (intravenous) methods; enteral (alimentary tract) methods, via mouth, nasogastric tube, gastrostomy.

Some patients in surgical wards will have very few problems related to nutrition and hydration. You should, however, always remember that any surgery is likely to disrupt both the patient's usual pattern of eating and drinking, and increase the need for nutrients.

Mrs Fellows, admitted for an operation on her varicose veins, is adequately hydrated and has been following the dietary advice she was given in the Outpatient Clinic and has managed to lose some weight. She is able to eat and drink normally on the day she is admitted but on the following day is allowed nothing at all by mouth for 4 hours prior to surgery. When she returns from theatre she is rather sleepy but is allowed to take fluids as soon as she feels able to sit up in bed. Later in the evening she has a light meal.

Mrs Fellows is well nourished and well hydrated before she has surgery. She only spends about 8 hours without food and fluid and is soon able to compensate for this.

Peter West's situation is rather different. The condition he is suffering from, peptic ulceration, is associated with poor eating habits, particularly irregular meals. Part of the treatment therefore requires that Peter should make changes in his lifestyle; for example, he should take regular meals and avoid spicy foods and alcohol. Peter needs to understand this and then, if given adequate help and support, will feel that he can make the major contribution towards restoring his own health (see also Chapter 3).

Elimination

Elimination is the process by which waste products are excreted from the body. The majority of waste products are eliminated in urine and faeces but some are excreted via the skin in sweating and during respiration.

Approximately 1,500 millilitres of urine is passed by an adult in 24 hours; defaecation may occur 3 times a day or 3 times a week. It is important that the nurse establishes what is the usual pattern for the patient.

Most people consider elimination to be a very private bodily function and therefore find it an embarrassing subject to discuss with hospital staff. Lack of privacy in hospital may also be a cause of problems with bladder or bowels; for example most patients find it difficult to use a bedpan, or commode in the ward area, even when well screened from other patients.

Micturition

Dysuria
Difficult or painful micturition.

Common problems of micturition may include poor urinary output, incontinence of urine, dysuria, frequency of micturition, retention of urine, or haematuria (blood in the urine).

If a patient complains of any of these problems the nurse should make a careful assessment of the situation by asking tactful questions. It is usual to record the fluid balance so that intake and output and their relationship may be assessed. The problems are sometimes related directly to the surgery, e.g. trauma to the bladder or urethra in pelvic or abdominal surgery; or retention of urine due to pain or lack of privacy. In other cases the problem may be a symptom of an underlying condition and tests may be necessary to diagnose this (e.g. urine tests, intravenous pyelogram, cystoscopy).

Defaecation

In view of individual variations, a careful assessment of bowel function is needed if a patient appears to have problems related to this. Tactful questioning about bowel habit is usually part of patient assessment in surgical wards for several reasons:

— To try to maintain 'normal' bowel function by keeping to the patient's own routine if possible, e.g. if a patient takes bran at breakfast, this should continue if not contra-indicated.
— For abdominal and pelvic operations, an empty bowel is usually required (if the patient is constipated, a mild laxative or 2 glycerine suppositories will usually ensure the bowel is emptied).
— Changes in bowel habit may indicate disease of the gastro-intestinal tract.

Melaena Black, tarry faeces due to the presence of altered blood.

Common problems related to bowel function may include constipation, diarrhoea, rectal bleeding, melaena or paralytic ileus.

You may work on a surgical unit which is entirely devoted to dealing with these prob-

lems but they may also occur in general
surgical wards.

Mr Reynolds is admitted to hospital because
he has complained of a change in bowel habit
and rectal bleeding. A manual examination
has revealed a mass in his rectum. It is necessary for the doctor and nurses to tactfully
discuss this with Mr Reynolds although he
finds it embarrassing (Chapter 3). In order for
the diagnosis to be confirmed, a barium enema
and later a biopsy of the tumour (via a sigmoidoscope) will be required.

Pre-operative period
Prior to these investigations it is necessary to
clear the bowel completely of faeces. This is
achieved by giving laxatives, enemas and finally at least one rectal washout. This is necessary so that the barium can pass into the bowel
for the X-ray procedure and so that good vision
can be obtained through the sigmoidoscope.

In Mr Reynolds' case it is necessary to repeat
this preparation after the investigations to ensure a good view for the surgeon and so that
faecal matter is not present to contaminate the
operation site. Dietary restrictions may also be
used to achieve this aim. Practice may vary but
it is usual to restrict fibre in the diet to reduce
the bulk of faeces. In some units a liquid, low
residue diet, containing all the essential
nutrients can be supplied. The dietician will
give advice so that each individual is given
adequate nourishment.

Because Mr Reynolds has lost weight prior
to admission to hospital and will have to receive bowel preparation for several days, it is
agreed that he should commence a liquid diet.
The dietician is consulted and provides a com-
mercially made liquid diet which will give Mr

Reynolds the nutrients he needs and is high in calories and protein.

Mr Reynolds' main preoccupation before his operation is with the stoma which will be formed during the procedure. All the nursing staff need to be aware of Mr Reynolds' concerns, although the stoma care nurse will probably deal with most of the patient's questions.

Post-operative period

When Mr Reynolds returned to the ward from the operating theatre, he had a drainable, clear plastic bag over his colostomy. There was a small amount of blood-stained fluid in the bag and staff nurse explained to the nurses that it was very important to record and report the amount and type of drainage via the colostomy. She also explained the importance of observing the colour and size of the stoma, especially noting any oedema or discolouration.

Mr Reynolds was not able to eat or drink and fluids were therefore administered through the central venous and intravenous lines which had been inserted in theatre. He had a nasogastric tube which was allowed to drain into a bag and was also aspirated every 4 hours to ensure that his stomach remained empty. Mr Reynolds needed the nasogastric tube for 4 days after his operation because he developed a paralytic ileus and it was not until the fourth post-operative day that the bowel began to work. He was then able to start taking fluids by mouth in gradually increasing amounts. The intravenous infusion was removed when he was able to take fluids without feeling nauseated.

An accurate record of Mr Reynolds' fluid intake and output was kept. Monitoring of his circulatory state via the central venous pressure line was not required after the first 24 hours and the line was therefore removed. The urinary catheter was not removed until the fourth day when Mr Reynolds was able to walk to the toilet with the help of the nurse.

On the 5th post-operative day Mr Reynolds became very distressed and eventually admitted to the nurse who was caring for him that his 'water works' were the source of his concern. She discovered that he had urinary frequency and it was decided that a specimen of urine should be sent to the bacteriology laboratory to discover whether he had a urinary tract infection.

The stoma care nurse visited Mr Reynolds later in the day and demonstrated to him how to change the colostomy appliance. He admitted that this was the first time he had really looked at the stoma and that he found the appearance and the smell rather offensive. The stoma care nurse was therefore careful to show no revulsion when changing the bag and explained to Mr Reynolds that the faecal fluid passing through the colostomy was not a permanent feature and that when he recommenced solid food the colostomy would produce more formed faeces. She encouraged him to try a small amount of soft food and to take nourishing foods such as soups. Mr Reynolds admitted that he had been afraid to eat or drink because of the possible effects on his bowel and bladder.

Rehabilitation and discharge

Diet and Fluids
Mr Reynolds was encouraged to take plenty of fluids orally (up to 2 litres per day) including nourishing substances and to gradually increase his diet until it was equivalent to his usual intake at home. He was weighed to ensure that he was beginning to regain some of the weight he lost pre-operatively. The stoma care nurse encouraged him not to avoid foods

but to monitor their effect on the colostomy action.

Bladder

The laboratory report showed that Mr Reynolds had a urinary tract infection and antibiotics were prescribed to treat this. He was encouraged to resume a normal fluid intake and not to restrict fluids because his bladder felt uncomfortable. He began to feel more comfortable after 24 hours' treatment with antibiotics and also admitted that he found it easier to pass urine in the privacy of the toilet than he did in the ward.

Stoma Care

The stoma care nurse carefully measured the size of the stoma and agreed with Mr Reynolds the type of bag he would like to wear. She taught both Mr and Mrs Reynolds the skills they needed to care for the stoma:

1   How to prepare the equipment.
2   Cleaning and drying the skin.
3   Application of a non-drainable bag with a protective flange attached.
4   Disposal of bags and cleansing materials.
5   How to obtain and store equipment.

Mr and Mrs Reynolds, the stoma care nurse and the ward sister agreed the day on which Mr Reynolds would go home. It was arranged that he would take a few days' supply of stoma bags with him and he was given a list of equipment he would require. His wife took this to their General Practitioner to obtain a prescription to ensure a continued supply (he does not have to pay for this). The stoma care nurse arranged that she would visit Mr Reynolds when he had been home 48 hours but gave him her telephone number in case he needed help before then. Mr and Mrs Reynolds both felt more secure about his homecoming once these arrangements were made.

1 Why is it important that all patients are well nourished prior to surgery? What factors would you take into consideration when assessing a patient's nutritional status?

2 What is a paralytic ileus? What actions are usually taken post-operatively to avoid this condition?

3 Choose a patient who is to undergo abdominal or pelvic surgery. Why may this patient develop bladder problems post-operatively? What nursing actions can be taken:
   (a) to avoid these problems?
   (b) to assist the patient if they occur?

FURTHER READING

Breckman, B. 1981. *Stoma Care: A Guide for Nurses, Doctors and Other Health Care Workers* Beaconsfield: Beaconsfield Publications.

Hamilton-Smith, S. 1972. *Nil by Mouth*. London: RCN.

Nutrition and Health. 1980. *Nursing*, 1st series, No. 11.

Nutrition and Illness. 1980. *Nursing*, 1st series, No. 12.

Wright, L. 1974. *Bowel Function in Hospital Patients*. London: RCN.

7

Skin and healing, temperature regulation, hygiene and comfort

Before reading this chapter you would find it helpful to revise the anatomy and physiology of:

1 Skin and wound healing
2 Temperature regulation.

Skin and Healing

An intact skin protects the internal structures from water loss and assists in temperature regulation. When skin integrity is interrupted by surgery, the wound provides a means for bacteria to enter, so precautions need to be

The skin

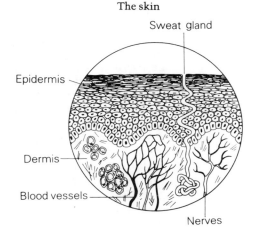

taken in the pre- and post-operative periods to prevent this occurrence.

Skin has the ability to repair itself, depending upon the size of the wound. Stress reduces the body's ability to heal and thus needs to be minimized. Continuous pressure on a skin surface represents a risk of pressure sore development. It is the nurse's responsibility to prevent pressure sores developing by relieving pressure at least 2 hourly, by alternating the patient's position.

If the wound is clean cut and free from debris, e.g. a surgical wound, the edges can be held together by internal and external sutures and primary healing takes place. Blood fills the space and clots, capillaries grow into the clot and form granulation tissue. Fibrous tissue replaces this, the capillaries heal and contract down over a period of months to leave a linear scar. A good supply of oxygenated blood is required for healing to occur, as is protein, vitamin C and rest. Anaemia and poor diet need to be corrected pre-operatively. Poor health, pre-existing disease (e.g. diabetes) and high stress levels can delay healing, as can haemorrhage or a collection of pus (abscess) in an infected wound.

Tissues should be able to support themselves unaided before sutures are removed. On the face and neck this usually takes 2−3 days as these areas heal quickly and early removal helps to reduce scarring. Abdominal sutures are usually left in situ for 7−10 days. Various types and patterns of sutures exist − unfortunately we do not have space to discuss them all here.

Skin preparation before surgery normally involves at least washing and may additionally include body hair removal to allow access to the operation site and also to reduce the risk of infection. It is especially important that no breaks in the skin occur during shaving as these act as routes for bacteria to enter. The exact extent of the area to be shaved varies according to the operation – it is best to check before shaving is commenced.

Wound care

Any break in skin continuity is a possible site for the entry of micro-organisms and needs to be treated with care to avoid infection. The natural protection for minor skin interruptions, e.g. grazes, scratches and puncture sites, is dried serous fluid and blood. This type of wound is best kept dry without a dressing.

The purpose of a dressing is to:

1   protect the wound from contamination by micro-organisms
2   absorb discharge which may hinder healing
3   support the wound and prevent movement of the wound edges.

There is a wide range of materials for wound dressing. All must be sterile. Dressings generally should be left undisturbed until it is time for suture removal unless:

1   the existing dressing is heavily soiled or wet with exudate
2   the patient complains of excess pain
3   an unexplained pyrexia exists
4   wound drains or tubes need attention.

Some surgeons may prefer the wound to be inspected after 48 hours and redressed, or a protective plastic skin sprayed on.

Surgical drains are placed by the surgeon into the wound and provide a route for the exit of blood or body fluids which would otherwise prevent healing. Usually made of rubber or soft polythene and draining into gauze or bags, they may be shortened or removed after 48 hours if the discharge is minimal. Drains are usually secured by a suture, and a sterile safety pin may be placed through the drain to prevent it retreating into the wound. When removing a drain for the first time, the suture must be removed, and the safety pin replaced about 1″ down the tube if it is to be shortened. This procedure is much easier if sterile gloves are worn.

Actual dressing techniques vary enormously. Check your local policy and the instructions you were given in lectures. You may find it useful to revise microbiology, the modes of spread of infection and methods of sterilization.

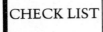

CHECK LIST

Aseptic Technique

General principles:
- All wounds should be treated aseptically (no touch technique).
- It is best if there is a separate room for dressings, and trolleys are kept solely for dressings.
- 2 nurses can perform a dressing more efficiently and cut down the length of time a wound is exposed and at risk and the number of times hands need to be washed.

Prepare the patient:
- Explain what is to happen and what the patient needs to do.
- If the procedure is long or the dressing painful analgesia may need to be given by injection ½–1 hour before the dressing. Alternatively an inhalational analgesic – a mixture of nitrous oxide and oxygen – can be inhaled before and during the procedure.

Prepare the area:
- Check that the proposed area for the procedure is clean, windows are closed and disturbances can be avoided.
- Ensure that there is a suitable place to dispose of soiled dressings.
- Collect equipment, including clean dressing trolley and sterile dressing materials and solutions. You may also need strapping, scissors, drainage bag, extra sterile instruments and/or a disposal bag for soiled dressings (depending on local policy and available equipment).

Prepare yourself:
- Ensure that you know what you are going to do.
- Do not do dressings if you have a cold, cough or any other infection.
- Wash hands thoroughly before commencing procedure.

Technique:
– Remove old dressing carefully – try not to disturb the wound. Soak dressing off if necessary.
– Observe the state of the old dressing, (e.g. the amount of drainage) and the wound.
– Cleanse the area if necessary – remember that the wound is best left dry as bacteria thrive in a moist, warm environment.
– Carry out any procedure which has been ordered (e.g. remove sutures, shorten drain).
– Renew dressing.
– Remember to report on the state of the wound.

Nursing responsibilities

When a patient is admitted the nurse should observe the skin to establish its normal colour and tone and identify any problem areas. Measures may be required to ensure that the patient's skin is in the best possible condition for healing to take place (e.g. general hygiene and nutrition are important).

Pre-operatively the nurse must check that the patient's skin is prepared as requested by the surgeon. During the operation the skin needs to be protected against diathermy burns.

Post-operatively the nurse should observe the wound for excess swelling (oedema) and haemorrhage and protect the wound from infection. Wound healing should be promoted by adherence to aseptic technique.

During the peri-operative period pressure sores should be prevented by regular changes of position.

NURSING CARE

Pre-operative period

Julie required minimal preparation for surgery. She had bathed and washed her hair during the evening before her admission to hospital.

As her temperature was raised (37.8°C) and her mouth felt dry, Julie's mother helped her to sponge her hands and face and clean her teeth before putting an operation gown on.

Peri-operative period

In the operating theatre a small area of her skin was shaved and cleaned with an antiseptic lotion once she was anaesthetized. When the operation was completed the small incision was sutured and a sealed dressing was applied. No drains were inserted.

Post-operative period

Following her return to the ward Julie's temperature was monitored every hour because it remained raised. Her wound was checked regularly for excess drainage but none was detected. Julie found it difficult to feel comfortable despite being given analgesia regularly. About 3 hours after her return to the ward she was helped to sit up in bed, propped up on pillows. At this time her intravenous infusion was removed and she seemed more relaxed but still complained of pain from her wound.

Two days after the operation the dressing was removed and the wound inspected; the suture line was intact and there was no excess redness or swelling. A wound swab was taken as Julie still had a pyrexia. The wound was then cleansed and redressed aseptically. Results from the wound swab revealed no infection and her temperature returned to within normal limits on the 3rd post-operative day.

Discharge

Before Julie went home the District Nurse was contacted and asked to redress the wound, and to remove the sutures on the 7th post-operative day. Julie was given dressing materials to take home. She was advised to bathe or shower daily and avoid straining her abdominal muscles and to see her General Practitioner to check that her recovery was progressing satisfactorily.

Temperature Regulation

The temperature regulation centre in the brain usually maintains the balance between heat production and loss. Any great variations in the normal range of body temperature (36°C to 37.5°C) represent a threat to cell functioning.

Measurement of body temperature provides useful information about a person's state of health – the most common sites for recording are the mouth and axilla. In the pre-operative period, a raised temperature may point to a contra-indication to surgery, e.g. infection. The patient's normal temperature range is established following admission and checked regularly in the early post-operative period.

In theatre the body is cooled to reduce the oxygen demand on the tissues, and during anaesthesia body temperature falls due to the effect of drugs. Following the operation the temperature usually rises by approximately 1°C due to the body's reaction to trauma. If the patient is shocked post-operatively, peripheral constriction makes the skin feel cold to the touch and the temperature recorded in the axilla may not represent the core temperature – post-operative recordings are more accurate if taken in the mouth. All post-operative temperature rises should be considered as being due either to chest problems, wound infection, urine infection, deep vein thrombosis or the introduction of bacteria during transfusion, until proved otherwise. It is therefore important to report all post-operative pyrexias.

NURSING CARE

Pre-operative period
When he was admitted to the ward, Mr Reynolds' temperature was recorded orally at

36.8°C. Throughout the pre-operative period it remained within normal limits.

Post-operative period
Immediately post-operatively his temperature fell to 35.8°C. Warmed blood was transfused to counteract shock and an extra blanket was placed around him.

After his return to the ward Mr Reynolds' temperature rose slowly until it reached 37°C. On the first post-operative morning his temperature was above normal limits (37.8°C). His skin was very pink and felt warm to touch and he complained of 'feeling hot and sweaty'. The extra blankets were removed and after a bedbath his skin felt cooler. His wounds were examined for signs of possible infection but they appeared quite satisfactory.

By the following morning Mr Reynolds was apyrexial and although his temperature was recorded every four hours for the next five days it remained within normal limits.

Hygiene

Regular performance of good hygiene practices helps to promote healthy skin, teeth and hair. The practice of personal hygiene is an almost automatic daily activity.

These normally private functions can assume unusually large proportions if illness limits a person's capacity for self care. Surgery may alter a person's hygiene needs, body secretions may dry up and form crusts requiring removal, especially if artificial tubes are inserted, e.g. catheters, nasogastric and endotracheal tubes.

It is important that the individual's normal hygiene practices are established and maintained where possible, and that the nurse does not impose her own values on others. There are social, cultural and spiritual aspects to hygiene which the nurse needs to be aware of so that people are not offended. If usual hygiene practices are not considered to be adequate then the nurse may need to explain tactfully what is required.

When admission to hospital is planned, people often purchase new or more luxurious items from the wide range of commercial hygiene products available. The performance of hygiene functions can be relaxing in themselves, and can provide a sense of security in the knowledge that one is socially acceptable. If the nurse can assist or provide hygiene measures in a sensitive manner, this may enhance the patient's personal comfort.

Comfort

The feeling of comfort is basic to a sense of well-being, but it is difficult to define and is often most notable in its absence. There are physical and psychological aspects to comfort and it cannot be considered in isolation from anxiety, pain (Chapter 3), position, rest and sleep (Chapter 8). Comfort is also related to environmental factors; noise, light and temperature. Due to the abstract and individual nature of comfort, the nurse will have to rely on the patient to tell her if he is uncomfortable, and whether any action taken has increased or decreased comfort. Discomfort is easier to ignore if the person is occupied, and appears worse when attention is focused solely upon it. Patients awaiting investigations or surgery may find it helpful to keep occupied, by reading or watching television.

For some people security and comfort can be derived from being able to anticipate events, for others ward routine can be a source of distress. It has been found that well-informed patients are less anxious and the nurse can help by explaining what is likely to happen in the pre-, peri- and post-operative periods.

Patients undergoing surgery sometimes find talking to a spiritual counsellor provides psychological comfort, even if they do not usually practise a religion.

Clothing can affect personal comfort. Whilst in hospital patients are encouraged to wear nightclothes. This may be a source of embarrassment; people do not usually meet for social or business purposes dressed in this way. For others the wearing of nightclothes may be contrary to their normal practice. It is easy for hospital staff to forget that patients may feel awkward or self-conscious at first.

The identification of the cause of discomfort is critical if nurses are to promote patient ease and comfort. Sensitivity of approach is a nursing skill required to help a tense and worried person feel more comfortable. As a junior nurse new to the surgical ward you are in a good position to understand how uncomfortable a person can feel in a strange place with unfamiliar people. Try to remember this feeling and more importantly, the things which helped you to relax – use this to help your patients to settle. They will have the added anxiety of the unknown prognosis, the possibility of pain and the feeling of powerlessness in a totally foreign environment.

NURSING CARE

Pre-operative period

Mr Reynolds arrived on the ward looking neat and well-groomed but ill at ease. His normal hygiene practices were established by the nurse who talked to him first and he was encouraged to continue with these. He was shown the location of the bathroom and toilets and the nurse discussed with him the extra hygiene measures which he would require to prepare him for surgery.

Mr Reynolds was also shown the ward day-room and introduced to other patients to help him settle down, but his anxiety about his condition prevented him from really relaxing.

On the morning of his operation a nurse helped Mr Reynolds to put on an operation gown after his bath and then encouraged him to rest in his freshly made up bed. Before giving his premedication, the nurse asked Mr Reynolds to empty his bladder. She then checked that the skin preparations were complete and asked him to remove his dentures. The effect of the premedication did help Mr Reynolds to relax for a short while prior to going to theatre.

Post-operative period

After Mr Reynolds' return to the ward post-operatively his position was changed every 2 hours to minimize the effects of pressure on his skin. Once he had regained consciousness his hands and face were sponged, he was given a mouthwash and changed into his own pyjamas.

During the first post-operative days a nurse performed catheter care 4 hourly to help prevent infection. Mr Reynolds was unable to take fluids orally and his mouth felt very dry. Therefore mouthwashes were given at least every two hours. The nurses helped with all his personal hygiene until he began to re-establish his independence.

All nursing and medical procedures were explained to Mr Reynolds and he was asked his preferences wherever possible. His position was changed at least every 2 hours and analgesia was offered regularly to promote relaxation and comfort.

1   Do any of your patients have problems maintaining personal hygiene? Find out how these problems are dealt with.
2   Find out the main factors on your surgical ward which help or hinder patient comfort.
3   Which measures for controlling body temperature are most commonly used on your ward?
4   Identify and explain which patients are most at risk of pressure sore development. Which sites are most at risk?
5   Find out if there are any special skin preparations ordered for patients on your ward and the reasons for these.
6   Find out what is the policy on your ward for:
     i) inspecting and dressing infusion sites
     ii) inspecting and redressing surgical wounds.
7   Find out which method of suturing is most commonly used on your ward. Observe how the sutures are removed and if you feel able to, practise their removal under supervision.

FURTHER READING

Boore, J. 1978. *A Prescription for Recovery*. London: RCN.

Hayward, J. 1975. *Information – A Prescription against Pain*. London: RCN.

Hunt, J. 1974. *The Teaching and Practice of Surgical Dressing in Three Hospitals*. London: RCN.

Royal Marsden Hospital, 1984. *Manual of Clinical Policies and Procedures*. London: Harper & Row.

8 Activity, sleep and rest

In the healthy person, there is normally a balance between activity and rest, ensuring that the individual has enough energy for daily life. However, the need for energy is increased by stress or illness, necessitating a corresponding increase in the amount of rest required. The individual's powers of recovery can be impaired by physical and mental exhaustion, as there are no reserves of energy to overcome the crisis. If the lack of energy is not remedied, the excess stress on the body can ultimately lead to prolonged illness and possible death.

Activity and Mobility

The activity level of an individual can be an indicator of his state of health. There are wide variations in the level of activity people accept as normal, however, so it is important to establish their usual pattern before making inferences. People whose mood is high are frequently over-active (although the activity may be purposeless), whereas a person whose mood is low may be apathetic and reluctant to move.

People are now being encouraged to take more exercise to promote health. Physical activity assists body function by improving circulation and muscle tone; exercise promotes deeper breathing and helps to prevent stasis in the gastro-intestinal tract. Physical exercise is most effective if taken 'little and often', avoiding strain and fatigue (although recently more active hobbies such as jogging and aerobics have become popular). Moderate exercise, for example walking and swimming, is thought to help prevent heart disease and should be encouraged in all age groups.

Activity can also help a person to relax both mentally and physically. Active hobbies provide physical occupation allowing the mind a break from other pressures, while hobbies requiring concentration can also divert the mind as well as preventing boredom and providing mental stimulation.

Ill health can reduce the individual's ability to move due to motor or nervous problems. Movement can also be limited by the body in order to protect itself from further harm, e.g. the pain from a twisted ankle prevents mobility, thus allowing the inflamed tissues to rest and heal.

Pain, or the fear of pain, can restrict mobility especially after surgery, when patients tend to lie still, keeping their whole body stiff regardless of the site of the pain or surgery. This natural protective reaction needs to be discouraged after surgery to avoid the complications of immobility. These are: joint stiffness, poor posture, muscle contractures, pressure sores, venous thrombosis and constipation. These problems can be avoided if the nurse explains to the patient why it is important to move, and assists the patient to move with the minimum of discomfort.

NURSING CARE

Pre-operative period

When Julie was first admitted to the ward she found it very difficult to rest comfortably due to the pain she was experiencing. Her mother said that she was normally a physically active girl, enjoying sports and walking, who usually fell asleep with no difficulty and slept soundly for 7–8 hours. However, Julie was now tired and miserable because of her pain and lack of sleep during the night prior to her admission. She said that the pain was a little better after the pethidine she had been given and she was able to rest quietly while she waited to be taken to theatre.

Post-operative period
Initially, after the operation, Julie was reluctant to move around because of pain from her wound. She was given analgesia and assisted by the nurses to change her position in bed. On the following morning both the nurses and the physiotherapist explained to Julie the importance of moving around. She was assisted to stand upright and walk to a chair. She was able to take analgesia orally and once her pain was controlled, she became more willing to move and adopt a less tense position.

Julie was given help to increase her level of mobility while in hospital and advice on how to return gradually to her former activities in the future.

Posture
The ability to alter body position is essential for the maintenance of normal body alignment. Poor posture can lead to problems, such as curvature of the spine, and can impair lung function. Incorrect positioning of limbs can lead to loss of function and contractures.

Under anaesthesia, neuromuscular control is lost and poor positioning of limbs in the peri-operative period can lead to a temporary loss of function if nerves have been pinched. It is important that all limbs are fully supported in a neutral position while the patient is anaesthetized.

Prolonged periods of time in one position can impair circulation and nerve supply, predisposing to pressure sore development. If a patient cannot change position at will, the nurse becomes responsible for doing it for him. The nurse's knowledge of various positions (see list below) will allow her to choose the position which will help the patient most.

Positions used in nursing

Name	*Description*

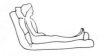

UPRIGHT — Sitting erect with support, e.g. backrest, pillows. Tendency to slip down – use footrest/tip bed to avoid this.
Uses: aids breathing.

ORTHOPNOEIC — Extended upright – leaning forward with arms resting on bedtable.
Uses: aids breathing.

SEMI-UPRIGHT — Resting back on pillows.
Uses: comfort, relaxation.

LATERAL LEFT/RIGHT — Lying on side, both arms facing forwards. Tendency to roll over if unsupported.
Uses: Relief of pressure, giving enema.

SEMI-PRONE — Lying partly on side and front – 1 arm flexed in front, 1 arm flexed behind – gives stability. Top knee more flexed than the other.
Uses: Unconsciousness, comfort/sleep.

RECOVERY — Exaggerated semi-prone – 1 arm flexed, 1 behind body along back.
Uses: Unconsciousness, relaxation.

PRONE — Lying on front, head to one side – use pillow under chest, arms flexed or straight by side.
Uses: Relief of pressure, injured spine, drainage of secretions.

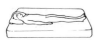

RECUMBENT/
DORSAL

Lying on back with knees straight or slightly flexed.
Uses: Comfort, relaxation, examination of abdomen, contra-indicated if chest problems.

TRENDELENBURG Head lower than trunk.
Uses: Shock, vaginal bleeding.

Sleep

Sleep can be defined as a period of reduced consciousness usually occurring at night, during which most body functions are slow or inactive. The exact function of sleep is unproven, but it is believed to be important in the maintenance of health and body repair. Some theorists dispute the need for sleep, while others insist a regular amount of sleep (the average being between 6 and 9 hours per night) is essential.

The effects of sleep deprivation appear to reduce mental and physical functioning. Sleeplessness can lead to feelings of listlessness, irritability and aggression. Prolonged hallucinations may occur. The body may attempt to make up for sleep lost at night by naps in the day, which can sometimes disturb the body's natural rhythm. It appears that a few extra hours of uninterrupted sleep can remedy the situation.

Two types of sleep occur during the sleep cycle. The first part involves a slowing down of brain waves. Approximately one hour after the onset of sleep, rapid eye movements beneath the closed lids occur (termed 'paradoxical sleep'), usually lasting about twenty minutes. A period of deep sleep with no eye movements ('orthodox sleep') follows. This cycle repeats itself approximately every 90 minutes. People wake more easily during the light paradoxical sleep, and take longer to fall into the more restful deeper orthodox sleep, especially if they are under stress or in an unfamiliar environment.

People who are ill often sleep more than usual. In this way the body reduces the demand for energy and reserves some for repair. Florence Nightingale considered lack of sleep to be an unnecessary additional discomfort for the sick and stressed the importance of environmental factors – some within and others outside the control of the nurse.

Patients often comment upon lack of sleep whilst in hospital. Sleep may be difficult to achieve and for some people a different bed in a strange environment surrounded by unfamiliar people and noises makes sleep impossible. The nurse may help promote sleep by reducing anxieties if possible and generally providing comfort – re-arranging pillows or adjusting the backrest. Other techniques for promoting sleep involve learning to control minds and bodies, for example by meditation, so that sleep can occur if possible.

Sleeping tablets are not always the solution as they upset the normal rhythm of sleep and people may become dependent upon them.

Rest and relaxation

Rest involves the cessation of action and freedom from worry. Like sleep, its function appears to be energy-saving and restorative. Unlike sleep, rest does not involve an alteration in conscious level. There are both physical and mental dimensions to rest; a change of activity or focus can itself be restful in states of ill health. In hospital it is not easy to rest. Anxiety regarding proposed surgery is natural and cannot be forgotten. Recreational pursuits may be helpful in directing attention from the main area of concern.

In order for patients to relax, they must feel secure and able to trust those caring for them. Trust takes time to develop and is not always possible in the short time available for pre-operative preparation. The nurse must use her communication skills to help the patient feel at ease.

While in hospital the responsibility for certain decisions is removed from the patient, e.g. what to wear, when to get up. For some people, this freedom from decision-making can help relieve pressures and may promote rest. For others, this loss of control can be a source of anxiety. Isolated from their normal environment and support network, some people find it almost impossible to relax. You should try to find out and, wherever possible adopt, the person's usual method of relaxation. It may also be possible to promote rest by teaching some specific relaxation technique, e.g. deep breathing, yoga.

As a junior nurse you may not feel able to assist the patient to rest or sleep – especially if you are not feeling fully at ease yourself! Do not be afraid to admit this and get help from others with more experience. Remember how you feel and what makes you relax – try to pass this on to your patients. A smile and a friendly gesture, a touch or holding a hand, can be an enormous help to patients.

HISTORY

Mrs Fellows had been finding it increasingly difficult to cope with her usual activities due to her aching legs and tiredness. After finishing work and her domestic chores she reported feeling 'fit for nothing except watching TV with my feet up'. Mrs Fellows also admitted to the nurse that she was a 'bit of a worrier' and found it hard to relax.

Pre-operative period

The nurse discussed with Mrs Fellows the importance of taking short walks, not sitting with her legs crossed and the continued wearing of support hose in the pre-operative period. Mrs Fellows was referred to the physiotherapist for teaching and practice of leg exercises before the operation.

The night before her operation Mrs Fellows was prescribed a sedative to help her relax and sleep because she admitted that she felt very nervous. After a milky drink she settled and slept until woken by the nurses for a cup of tea at 6.30 a.m. This was the last drink Mrs Fellows was allowed prior to her operation. After the final pre-operative preparations were completed, a premedication was given at 11.00 a.m. and Mrs Fellows dozed comfortably until she was escorted to theatre.

Post-operative period

When she returned to the ward the foot of the bed was elevated to tip the bed to an angle of 45°. A bedcradle was placed so that it relieved the weight of the bedclothes from her legs. As she woke up she was encouraged to move around in bed and wiggle her toes. Later she was assisted to sit up in bed.

On the morning after her operation her wounds were inspected and the bandages replaced by elastic stockings. She was then helped out of bed and assisted to walk around.

Discharge

Mrs Fellows was told that she could go home but that she should continue her leg exercises and avoid standing in one position for long periods. She was also advised that she should continue to try to reduce weight and should not return to her work (which involved standing all the time) until she had been seen in the Outpatient Clinic in six weeks time. The District Nurse would remove her sutures in seven days time.

ACTIVITIES

1 Identify the causes of limited mobility in the post-operative period. What nursing actions may be selected to deal with the problems?
2 Select a patient and ask him whether his surgery affected his normal pattern of rest and sleep.
3 Identify factors in your ward which help or hinder a patient's rest and sleep.

FURTHER READING

Henderson, V. 1969. *Basic Principles of Nursing Care*. Switzerland: ICN.
Osward, I. 1974. *Sleep*. Harmondsworth: Penguin.
Nightingale, F. 1969. *Notes on Nursing: What It Is and What It Is Not*. New York: Dover.
Sleep and Comfort. 1980. *Nursing*, 1st series, No. 20.
Mobility. 1984 and 1985. *Nursing*, 2nd series, Nos. 31, 32 and 33.

9 Rehabilitation and discharge from the surgical ward

Restoration of health

One of the aims of surgical care is to restore the patient to his previous level of functioning. The degree to which this can be achieved varies. In some cases, the aim of nursing care may be to promote adaptation to the new situation, as previous function has not been restored completely.

Julie had her appendix removed. She was discharged from hospital within a week and by that time, could carry out the majority of her normal activities. She had a wound that was still uncomfortable and restricted some of her movements, but once the sutures were removed, the discomfort would gradually decrease. She would be able to return to school within 2 or 3 weeks, but would be advised not to take part in any sports for several weeks after that. The appendix does not have any function in man (i.e. it is a vestigial organ) and therefore its removal would make no difference to Julie's normal activities once she had recovered from the operation itself.

For patients who undergo major procedures, rehabilitation is a longer process. The patient may need to adapt to living in a new way (e.g. Mr Reynolds' stoma) or without a particular organ or a limb which will make considerable alterations in lifestyle (e.g. an amputation).

Some patients may also have surgery which causes them fear, anxiety or grief (e.g. surgery for malignant conditions, disfiguring surgery to face, mastectomy).

A team approach is needed for the rehabilitation process. In most surgical units this team includes the specialist nurses, the physiotherapist and the occupational therapist.

Specialist nurses

Many health authorities employ nurses in specialist roles to care for patients with particular needs. The stoma care nurse has already been mentioned in this context. Specialist nurses have particular expertise in one field of nursing, usually in an area where the patient and family need teaching and support at home as well as in hospital. The stoma care nurse, for example, first meets patients in hospital but continues to visit them when they go home. This ensures continuity of care between hospital and home and gives the patient confidence to cope with a new situation.

Another type of specialist nurse deals solely with patients who have had a mastectomy. These patients, apart from fearing the surgical procedure and the effects of malignant disease, often have severe psychological problems after surgery. Such problems are usually related to grief and concern about loss of femininity and a feeling of disfigurement. Pre-operative counselling and support are as important as physical care and some hospitals provide a specialist nurse to help the patient deal with both the physical and psychological problems. This nurse may first see the patient in the Outpatient Clinic prior to admission and usually offers a counselling service for as long as necessary post-operatively. A psychologist or psychiatrist may also be involved in this service.

Continuing care

Palliative A surgical procedure which relieves symptoms but is not curative.

A few patients in surgical wards are found to have inoperable conditions or conditions for which only palliative surgery can be performed. This is sometimes the case in advanced malignant disease. Some of these patients will continue to be nursed in a surgical ward, some will be able to go home and others to a hospice for care. The decision will depend upon the condition and preference of the patient and the support and facilities available.

The aim of care is always to ensure the patient's physical and psychological comfort until death occurs. If the patient has a great deal of pain this is likely to be the most important aspect of nursing care and will involve using skill and imagination, for example in assisting the patient with activities, in lifting and positioning. Analgesia is usually given regularly to ensure that pain is kept under control at all times.

If there is someone willing and able to care for them, patients usually go home. The patient and family are then helped and supported by their General Practitioner and community nurses. In some areas there is a specialist home nursing service for the terminally ill and this is sometimes part of the services of a hospice (these are usually called Continuing Care or MacMillan nurses).

Discharging patients from surgical wards

It is important that adequate pre-discharge assessment takes place to ensure that patients do not go home to situations where they are unable to cope or inadequately supported. Ideally this type of assessment begins when the patient is admitted to hospital so that there is adequate time for planning if special arrangements have to be made prior to the patient going home.

The type of information required for discharge planning:

Type and condition of housing, e.g. stairs to be climbed; whether there is a bathroom and indoor toilet.

Family (or other) support available. Do they live in the house or visit? What do they usually do for the patient?

Aids already provided (if any).

Does the patient receive any services, e.g. district nurse; home help; Meals on Wheels?

This information and knowledge will help the nurse and the patient to decide how the patient will manage at home and whether extra assistance may be needed. Advice about any adaptations required will usually be given by the physiotherapist or occupational therapist and the patient may be taken on a home visit to assess his needs (e.g. amputees may need several aids). Information about services available in the community is usually sought from the medical social worker.

A few days before discharge is expected, any services required are arranged and any drugs, dressings and appliances (e.g. Mr Reynolds' stoma equipment) are ordered. These are available on prescription when the patient is at home but it is usual to give several days' supplies to patients in case they are unable to obtain a prescription immediately.

It is essential that relatives have adequate warning so that they can make arrangements for the patient's homecoming. Sister (or her deputy) will find out whether the patient requires an ambulance or hospital car to take him home. Many patients will have a family member who can collect them by car. This is often more comfortable for the patient and relieves the ambulance service. If the services of a district nurse are needed, she may be contacted by telephone or there may be a community liaison service in your hospital, in which case a member of the community nursing team will visit the ward and meet the patient. In addition a letter is usually written to the community nurse about the care the patient requires. Other people who need to be notified of the patient's discharge from hospital are the patient's General Practitioner and any specialist nurse who is involved in his care.

Some patients may not have friends or relatives able to give them support at home, or may live in unsuitable accommodation. They may therefore benefit from a period in a convalescent home if this can be arranged.

Nursing responsibilities

1   Help the patient to wash and dress in preparation for the journey.
2   Ensure the patient has all his belongings and help with packing if needed.
3   Ensure the patient has the following:
    appliances
    dressings
    drugs (with written instructions if necessary)
    completed forms/letters (e.g. for district nurse)
    appointment card (this may be sent to the patient later).
4   Ensure that the patient understands all information given and has no further queries.

In some surgical units, many patients are only in hospital for a day (e.g. Peter) or may be discharged very quickly after surgery (e.g. Mrs Fellows). However, the same principles apply to planning the discharge of these patients. The time for planning and making arrangements will be much shorter and therefore the nurse must ensure that she obtains adequate information from the patient (or family) on admission. Although these patients may have had smaller surgical procedures performed, they will require as much, or more, care at home because they are discharged earlier.

The aim of all these procedures is to ensure that no patient arrives home without the drugs or equipment needed or is left without adequate care and support.

HISTORY

Mr Brown took longer than is usual to recover from his hernia repair. His post-operative progress was complicated by a chest infection and he found it very difficult to regain his usual level of activity because his arthritis seemed worse after the operation and a day or two spent largely in bed.

When it was decided that Mr Brown would soon be fit to go home, sister contacted the warden of the flats in which he lived to discuss arrangements with her. The warden said that she would be able to call on Mr Brown at least once each day and explained that he had a bell to ring to call her if he felt unwell. She and sister agreed that Mr Brown would need additional help. The warden said that she would turn the heating on so that the flat would be warm and she would be there herself to welcome him home.

Sister then discussed the situation with Mr Brown and the medical social worker. It was agreed that sister would ask the district nurse to visit him to assess his mobility at home and give him help initially to bath. Mr Brown had already had his sutures removed and his wound was healed. The medical social worker said that she would request a home help for Mr Brown and also Meals-on-Wheels several times a week.

Although Mr Brown normally enjoys his independence and likes his flat, he admitted to sister that he felt a little apprehensive about going home. He felt that although his chest infection was better he was not really as active as he would like to be. He said he was pleased about the help offered to him but stressed to sister that he regarded the need for help as temporary: 'Until I'm really back on my feet again'.

It was arranged that Mr Brown would go home by ambulance and transport was also ordered to bring him for his Outpatient appointment in four weeks time. His General Practitioner was notified by telephone of his impending discharge and promised to visit him within a couple of days.

Mr Brown left the ward taking with him letters for the district nurse and his General Practitioner, an Outpatient appointment card and a supply of drugs (to treat his chronic bronchitis). He said he would miss having company day and night but was looking forward to returning home.

ACTIVITIES

1 Next time you admit a patient use the information you gain about his home circumstances and your knowledge about the operation he is to undergo to try and decide what care he might need when he leaves hospital. Try to make a plan for arranging this patient's discharge from hospital.

2 Choose a patient who has had major surgery and list all the arrangements that will need to be made for his discharge home. Who can help you to plan this and what services will this patient need?

FURTHER READING

Charles-Edwards, A. 1983. *The Nursing Care of the Dying Patient.* Beaconsfield: Beaconsfield Publications.

Plant, J. A. & Devlin, B. 1978. Planned early discharge of surgical patients. *Nursing Times*, Occasional Paper 74 (7), 25–28.

Roberts, I. 1975. *Discharged from Hospital.* London: RCN.

Tait, A., *et al.* 1982. Improving Communication Skills. *Nursing Times*, 78 (51), 2181–2184.

Wilson-Barnett, J. & Fordham, M. 1982. *Recovery from Illness.* Chichester: John Wiley and Sons.

10 Summary: planning care for patients undergoing surgery

In order to relate theory to practice in this book, human activities have been divided up into concept groups and the nurse's responsibilities in the pre-, peri- and post-operative periods have been considered. This summary is intended to be an overview of the care a patient may receive whilst on a general surgical ward.

It is highly unlikely that any individual patient will actually receive all the care as planned in this summary, as each individual is unique, so care will be planned to suit particular needs and will be changed according to the response of the patient to the plan.

A high proportion of nursing actions on a surgical ward are directed towards the prevention of problems. To a junior nurse it may appear that surgical nursing is negative in its aims. The overall aim is in fact positive – to help patients to obtain most benefit from their surgery and ultimately to improve their level of health. The nurse's role in the care of patients throughout their stay in the surgical ward is crucial to the outcome of the operation.

The following summary of nursing responsibilities for the care of surgical patients may appear complex at first glance and impossible to remember. *Do not be overawed.* Think about what you are trying to achieve and things will eventually fit into place.

Admission

In an ideal situation, surgery is planned and patients are admitted to the ward prior to the operation so that they may be prepared physically and psychologically for their forthcoming operation. During this time the nurses can get to know the patient, and vice versa, and establish the patient's normal condition against which the post-operative state can be compared.

In certain situations this period of preparation has to be completed within *hours*, not days, due to the urgent nature of the patient's problem (e.g. Julie Smith's appendicitis). In each case the overall aims of nursing remain the same.

Aims of care on admission

1 To help the patient settle on the ward and feel at ease.
2 To establish a relationship with the patient based on trust and open communication.
3 To help the patient to understand the investigations and proposed surgery.
4 To establish the patient's base-line observations against which post-operative comparisons will be made.

Care during admission

1 Welcome the patient in a friendly manner and introduce yourself to him.
2 Show the patient to his bed and ask the patient to change into nightwear. Show him the location of the toilets, dayroom etc.
3 Collect the information required for nursing assessment in conversation with the patient and/or relative. Provide information about ward routines and procedures, visiting times and telephone numbers. Answer any questions the patient may have.

4 Perform base-line observations: temperature, pulse, respiratory rate, blood pressure, urinalysis. Check height and weight.
5 Check personal details are correct and securely attach an identity band.
6 Explain that the doctor will perform a medical assessment and obtain formal consent for operation later.
7 Introduce the patient to his neighbours and leave him to settle into the ward, but be available for discussion.
8 Complete nursing records.

Pre-operative period

Nursing responsibilities centre upon the prevention of potential complications.

Aims of care in the pre-operative period
1 To ensure that the patient is in the best psychological and physical condition for the operation.
2 To prepare the patient physically and psychologically to avoid or minimize the risk of post-operative complications.
3 To ensure the patient is correctly prepared for theatre at the right time with the documentation complete.

Care in the pre-operative period
1 Explain simply and briefly the procedures necessary to prepare the patient for his operation, giving details of the patient's role in these and the reasons for them.
2 Explain the procedures in the post-operative period and reasons for them. Show the equipment which will be in use.
3 Encourage the patient to ask questions and discuss any fears or worries. Offer the services of a minister of religion.
4 Ensure, whenever possible, that a familiar nurse prepares the patient. Check the

patient understands what is to happen before preparation commences. Allow the patient to participate as much as possible.

5 Request physiotherapist visits for pre-operative assessment and to teach post-operative breathing and leg exercises.

6 Ensure medical investigations have been ordered and completed before operation time.

On-going care

1 Provide light easily digested protein-rich diet until time for withdrawal of food.

2 Ensure fluid input approximately 2 litres daily.

3 Ensure a balance between activity and rest.

4 Encourage patient to practise deep breathing exercises.

5 Assist with daily living activities where required.

6 Continue to monitor vital signs to detect changes in patient's condition which would make surgery inadvisable.

Physical preparation

Day before operation

1 Ensure the skin is clean with a bath or shower.

2 If a pre-operative shave is indicated the patient may require assistance.

Night before

1 Try to ensure a good night's sleep.

2 Alleviate any anxiety if possible.

Operation day

1 Withdraw diet at least 6 hours before operation time.

2 Withdraw fluid at least 4 hours before operation time.

3 Ask patient to bath/shower, dress in clean operation gown and remove jewellery, prostheses, make up.

4 Return patient to freshly made bed and encourage to rest quietly.

Before giving pre-medication

1 Request the patient to empty his bladder. Test urine and report abnormalities.
2 Check the consent form has been signed and preparations completed.
3 Check that dentures and prostheses have been removed or jewellery covered with sticky tape.
4 Check that no food or drink has been consumed in the preceding 6 and 4 hours respectively.
5 Administer pre-medication as ordered (usually ½ to ¾ hour before operation time). Explain that the patient's mouth will become dry and he may feel sleepy. Ask the patient to remain in bed, leave him to rest but keep under observation.
6 Complete documentation ready for transfer to the care of the theatre staff. Collect medical notes, consent form, X-rays, nursing notes/charts/prescription sheet.

Peri-operative period

This period covers the time from the patient's transfer from the ward to the theatre until the patient returns to the ward. The exact point of the transfer of responsibility from the ward to the theatre staff varies. Some theatre staff take over on the patient's arrival in the theatre suite and keep the patient until he is fully recovered and conscious, while in other theatres the ward nurse remains with her patient until he is fully anaesthetized (in some cases the ward nurse assists the anaesthetist) and returns to collect the patient who is not fully conscious and still under the effect of the anaesthetic. *Check what the procedure is in your area.*

If the theatre is a long distance away from the ward, equipment may be taken from the ward on a post-operative tray or carried on the theatre trolley.

Aims of care

1 To ensure that the patient arrives comfortably and safely at the theatre at the agreed time.
2 To prepare the bed area for the post-operative period.
3 To ensure the patient returns to the ward in comfort and safety with the correct post-operative instructions for his continuing care.

Care in the peri-operative period

1 Inform patient quietly that he is to be transferred to theatre.
2 Perform checking procedure according to local policy. Check correct patient by using notes, identity band and verbal check with patient.
3 Ensure correct documentation accompanies patient (usually medical notes, X-rays, prescription chart, fluid chart).
4 Patient accompanied to theatre by a familiar ward nurse who may remain with him until fully anaesthetized.

After patient has left ward

1 Prepare bed area for patient's return. Place bed in a position for easy observation and access to oxygen and suction. Ensure emergency resuscitation equipment is nearby and in working order and that the emergency call system is working.
2 Collect any equipment which will be required, e.g. for care of intravenous infusions, nasogastric tubes, vomit bowl and tissues, bedcradle and cot sides.
3 Collect equipment to monitor vital signs and charts to record them on.

When collecting patient from theatre
The same nurse should collect her patient
wherever possible.

1 Check the patient's condition.
2 Obtain information from the theatre staff
  including details of operation performed,
  orders for post-operative fluid regime,
  management of nasogastric aspiration,
  wound drains.
3 Check oxygen and post-operative analgesia
  have been prescribed.
4 If the ward nurse is satisfied with the
  patient's condition she accepts him back
  into her care and escorts him quietly back
  to the ward ensuring his safety by maintaining the airway and close observation.

Post-operative period

This period commences when the ward nurse
returns to the ward with the patient. The
condition of the patient on transfer varies from
theatre to theatre and depends upon whether
or not the theatre has a recovery room where
patients recover from the immediate effects of
the anaesthetic. Check the procedure in your
area.

Aims of care
1 To prevent or detect promptly any complications occurring after surgery.
2 To restore maximum health and independence as soon as possible after surgery.

Care in the immediate post-operative period
1 Inform the patient of his return to the ward
  and of the procedures you are about to
  perform.
2 Transfer the patient to the prepared area.
  Place the patient in the semi-prone position. Use oro-pharangeal airway, oxygen

and suction as necessary to maintain the airway.

3 Check vital signs ½ hourly at first, reduce frequency when stable. Report abnormalities promptly.

4 Check wounds and drain sites for haemorrhage, record amount of drainage on fluid chart.

5 Regulate and monitor infusion, record fluid intake and output. Aspirate nasogastric tube if indicated.

6 Once conscious gradually elevate patient to upright position. Encourage him to alter position 2–4 hourly. Regular analgesia should relieve the pain which prevents the patient moving around freely and performing deep breathing exercises.

Continuing care

1 Keep patient informed of progress and of procedures.

2 Continue to monitor vital signs.

3 Record input and output. Oral fluids are introduced gradually until a normal level is reached.

4 Once bowel function returns diet is gradually re-introduced. Monitor bowel action – use commode or toilet when possible.

5 Continue skin and mouth care as required, encourage the patient to become independent when able.

6 Gradually increase mobility as indicated. Monitor pattern of sleep and try to provide undisturbed periods so that the patient can rest.

7 Leave wound dressings undisturbed unless leaking or problems suspected.

8 Shorten drains, remove sutures as instructed and redress the wound using aseptic technique.

Rehabilitation and Discharge

Aims of care

1 To ensure maximum fitness and independence is achieved.

2 To ensure a co-ordinated return to the community.

3 To ensure a follow-up appointment to evaluate the results of the surgery.

Care for discharge

Planning for discharge should commence on admission and include assessment of the home circumstances and support available.

1 Contact community nurses and other services if they are likely to be required. Make referral when indicated. Provide information for community staff.

2 Provide any dressing equipment needed for the early days after discharge.

3 Order a supply of the drugs the patient requires. (Further supplies can be obtained from the General Practitioner.)

4 Check that a medical discharge note explaining what operation the patient has had is sent to the General Practitioner. (A full medical summary may follow.)

5 Ensure that an Outpatient appointment is made either before discharge or sent to the patient at a later date.

6 Enquire whether the patient will require hospital transport home and to return to Outpatients (48 hours' notice is usually required).

7 Explain how to care for themselves when at home and who to contact if problems are experienced.

11 Conclusion

You may now also be leaving the surgical ward. We hope that you have enjoyed the experience and have been able to learn the principles of surgical nursing.

It is important that you achieve a sound knowledge base and feel confident in performing practical skills, which will also be useful in other areas of nursing. We hope that you have gained a good grounding to enable you to give a high standard of nursing care in the future and some understanding not only of what happens on the surgical ward but also the care which may be required by people leaving the ward, whatever their stage of recovery.

Remember that surgical care is a team effort and that you are a valued and important member of the team.

INDEX

NOTES

NOTES